Bariatric Cookbook
Mega Bundle

Gastric Sleeve Cookbook Stage 1   page 3

50 Delicious Herbal & Other Teas, Sugar Free Popsicles & Ice Treats, Broth Recipes You Can Enjoy in Stage 1 Post Weight Loss Surgery Rehabilitation

Gastric Sleeve Cookbook Stage 2   page 51

50 Delicious Protein Shakes & Smoothies, Soups and Puddings Recipes You Can Enjoy in Stage 2 Post Weight Loss Surgery Rehabilitation

Bariatric Cookbook Stage 3   page 121

70+ Delicious Breakfast, Sandwiches, Soups, Slow Cooking, Cold & Hot Snack and Desert Recipes You Can Enjoy in Stage 3 Post Weight Loss Surgery Rehabilitation

Bariatric Cookbook Stage 4   page 222

80 Delicious Breakfast, Lunch, Dinner, Snack and Desert Recipes You Can Enjoy in Stage 4 Post Weight Loss Surgery

Gastric Sleeve Cookbook Stage 1

50 Delicious Herbal & Other Teas, Sugar Free Popsicles & Ice Treats, Broth Recipes You Can Enjoy in Stage 1 Post Weight Loss Surgery Rehabilitation

Table of Contents

Introduction

Congratulations on successfully completing your gastric sleeve surgery! Your new body is going to look great! Now that your surgery is in the past, the hard task of recovery begins. In order to ensure that you recover well and that you maintain the healthy body, you desire you will have to ensure you follow a proper nutrition plan, and it needs to begin right now! Before you can understand how to move on it is vital that you first understand what it is that your body just went through.

What exactly is Gastric Sleeve Surgery & What does it entail?

Gastric Sleeve or Weight Loss Surgery is a procedure used to help people suffering from obesity to get back to a healthy stage in life by surgically assisting in their weight loss. During the surgery, a portion of the stomach is removed so as to get it smaller (gastric sleeve).

So, what happens now?

Post your operation; there are four main nutrition goals that you will need to follow. These goals include ensuring you consume the correct amount of protein as this will aid in minimizing the loss of muscle tissue and help to speed up the recovery process. Next would be for you to learn the steps of eating properly as this will assist you in staying healthy in the long run. Thirdly you will need to remember to remain hydrated, ensuring that you drink enough water will be vital to your recovery process. Finally, you will need to ensure that you get the proper nutrients in your body by using supplements for minerals, and vitamins as you won't be able to eat solid food for a while after your surgery.

There will be 4 main stages in terms of food and diet that you will go through post your surgery. Namely:

- Stage 1 – Consuming only Clear Liquids

- Stage 2 – Consuming Thicker Liquids & Smooth Foods
- Stage 3 – Consuming Soft Pureed Foods
- Stage 4 – Consuming Regular Foods

This Gastric Sleeve Cookbook will focus on Stage 1 of your post gastric sleeve surgery recovery process helping you to understand what you can eat. So, let's explore Stage 1 of the recovery process a bit more so that you can fully understand what is expected at this stage.

Stage 1 – Consuming only Clear Liquids

This stage generally encompasses the first 7 days after your surgery, however, in all cases, it may be different. In this stage of the recovery, it is recommended that you stick to a diet filled with clear liquids. Sticking to clear liquids will allow your body to heal without disruption from the foods that your stomach would need to digest. You will, of course, need to take it slowly at first, so it's recommended, to begin with trying to drink about two ounces of liquid at a time as often as every 30 minutes. After which based on how you feel you can slowly increase your intake to up to eight ounces per hour. It is important to note that eating or drinking may cause discomfort so try to drink slowly, sip and not gulp.

Remember hydration is vital in this stage of recovery so try to consume at least 48 ounces to 64 ounces of liquid per day.

Here are some Important Tips to Remember:

- Try to avoid drinks with too much sugar, caffeine or carbonation as they can disrupt the healing process by causing side effects.
- Be sure to sip and not gulp as drinking in small portions makes it better for your body to readjust.
- Drinking a lot of liquids is of utmost importance, recording your daily liquid intake may help you greatly in avoiding dehydration.

8

So now that you know a bit more about Gastric Sleeve Surgery let's explore a bit more about what exactly you can eat within this clear liquid the only stage. In this Gastric Sleeve Cookbook, you will be exposed to 50 simple yet tasty recipes that are all easy on the stomach. Without further ado, let's get started.

Herbal & Other Teas

Peppermint Tea

This tea is said to help with abdominal gas and bloating.

Preparation time: 37 minutes
Yield: 4 servings

Ingredients
- Peppermint Leaf (1/2 cup, dried)
- Water (4 cups, hot)

Directions
1. Set your water on to boil. Once boiling add in your peppermint leaves and remove from heat.
2. Cover and let rest for at least 5 minutes.
3. Strain, serve and enjoy

Macros per Serving & Nutrition Facts
- Calories 34.2
- Total Fat 0.0 g
- Carbohydrate 9.1 g
- Protein 0.1g

Pecan Tea

Yet another warm beverage is perfect for the early mornings.

Preparation Time: 20 minutes
Serving: 2

Ingredients
- Pecans (5 tablespoons, grounded)
- Cinnamon (1 tsp.)
- Water (1 cup)
Directions

1. Heat a cup of water in a saucepan and then stir in your remaining ingredients.
2. Serve hot.

Macros per Serving & Nutrition Facts
- Calories 40
- Total Fat 3.58 g
- Carbohydrate 1.4 g
- Protein 1.51 g

Ginger Tea

This tea has been known to help curb an upset stomach, nausea and even subdue vomiting.

Preparation time: 15 minutes
Yield: 2 serving

Ingredients
- Gingerroot (3 tsp., grated))
- Boiling Water (3 cups)

Directions
1. Combine your ingredients together and allow to rest, covered for at least 10 minutes.
2. Serve and Enjoy!

Macros per Serving & Nutrition Facts
- Calories 26.8
- Total Fat 0.0 g
- Carbohydrate 6.8 g
- Protein 0.1 g

Orange Vanilla Tea

Classic Orange tea with a hint of vanilla, for a surprise.

Preparation time: 11 minutes
Yields: 2.5 Cups

Ingredients
- Water (1/4 cup)
- Oranges (2, medium, peeled, sliced)
- Vanilla Extract (1/4 tsp.)

Directions
1. Pour all your ingredients into a saucepan and allow to come to a boil.
2. Remove from heat and let rest for about 5 minutes.
3. Strain, serve and enjoy!

Macros per Serving & Nutrition Facts
- Calories 60
- Total Fat 0.0 g
- Carbohydrate 14 g
- Protein 1g

Peanut Tea

Get something warm in the morning.

Preparation Time: 20 minutes
Serving: 2

Ingredients
- Peanut (5 tablespoons, grounded)
- Cinnamon (1 tsp.)
- Water (1 cup)

Directions
1. Heat a cup of water in a saucepan and then stir in your remaining ingredients.
2. Serve hot.

Macros per Serving & Nutrition Facts
- Calories 40
- Total Fat 3.58 g
- Carbohydrate 1.4 g
- Protein 1.51 g

Red Apple and Carrot Tea

This tea is best for chronic constipation. Make it and drink 1 glass daily for better results.

Preparation time: 6 minutes
Yield: 3 servings

Ingredients
- 1 cup red apples, peeled, chunks
- 2 carrots, sliced
- ½ cup lychee, seeded
- 2 cups water

Directions
1. Blend apples with carrots, lychee, and water.
2. Pour all your ingredients into a saucepan and allow to come to a boil.
3. Remove from heat and let rest for about 5 minutes.
4. Strain, serve and enjoy!

Macros per Serving & Nutrition Facts
- Calories 184
- Total Fat 0.0 g
- Carbohydrate 44.6g
- Protein 1g

Orange Carrot Tea

This recipe gives a rich blend of both orange and carrot. If you love a strong citrusy drink, you will love this!

Yields: 5 cups
Time Needed: 11 minutes

Ingredients
- Oranges (4, peeled, halved)
- Carrots (12 oz., diced)
- Water (4 Cups)

Directions
1. Pour all your ingredients into the Vitamix and secure the lid.
2. Pour all your ingredients into a saucepan and allow to come to a boil.
3. Remove from heat and let rest for about 5 minutes.
4. Strain, serve and enjoy!

Macros per Serving & Nutrition Facts
- Calories 93
- Total Fat 0.4 g
- Carbohydrate 22 g
- Protein 2.2g

Almond Tea

Begin your day with a splash of almond tea.

Serving: 2
Preparation Time: 20 minutes

Ingredients
- Almond Powder (5 tablespoons)
- Cinnamon (1 tsp.)

- Water (1 cup)

Directions
1. Heat a cup of water in a saucepan and then stir in your remaining ingredients.
2. Serve hot.

Macros per Serving & Nutrition Facts
- Calories 40
- Total Fat 3.58 g
- Carbohydrate 1.4 g
- Protein 1.51 g

Rooibos Tea

Packed with vitamin C, as well as other antioxidants and minerals, this tea aids immensely in the recovery process.

Preparation time: 30 minutes
Yield: 4 servings

Ingredients
- Rooibos (1/2 cup)
- Water (4 cups, hot)

Directions
1. Set your water on to boil. Once boiling add in your rooibos pieces and remove from heat.
2. Cover and let rest for at least 15 minutes.
3. Strain, serve and enjoy

Macros per Serving & Nutrition Facts
- Calories 1
- Total Fat 0.0 g
- Carbohydrate 0.1 g
- Protein 0 g

Chamomile Tea

This tea can be used as a natural sedative as it calms the nerves. It is also said to aid in the digestion process which makes it a brilliant option during stage 1 recovery.

Preparation time: 10 minutes
Yield: 2 servings

Ingredients
- Chamomile Flowers (2 tbsp.)
- Water (2 cups)

Directions
1. Set your water on to boil. Once boiling add in your chamomile and remove from heat.
2. Cover and let rest for at least 5 minutes.
3. Strain, serve and enjoy

Macros per Serving & Nutrition Facts
- Calories 1
- Total Fat 0 g
- Sodium 4.7 mg
- Carbohydrate 0.1 g
- Protein 0.0g

Lemon Balm Tea

This tea is great for relaxation.

Preparation time: 20 minutes
Yield: 5 servings

Ingredients
- Lemon Balm (1 cup)
- Water (5 cups)

- Lemon Zest (1 tbsp.)

Directions
1. Set your water on to boil. Once boiling add in your lemon balm, and zest then remove from heat.
2. Cover and let rest for at least 10 minutes.
3. Strain, serve and enjoy

Macros per Serving & Nutrition Facts
- Calories 13.3
- Total Fat 0 g
- Carbohydrate 3.6 g
- Protein 0.0g

Dandelion Tea

Here is a tea that works to cleanse your livers, and aids in bile production which is vital in the digestion process.

Preparation time: 10 minutes
Yield: 2 servings

Ingredients
- Dandelion Flowers (2 tbsp.)
- Water (2 cups)

Directions
1. Set your water on to boil. Once boiling add in your dandelion and remove from heat.
2. Cover and let rest for at least 5 minutes.
3. Strain, serve and enjoy

Macros per Serving & Nutrition Facts
- Calories 8
- Total Fat 0 g
- Carbohydrate 0.0 g
- Protein 0.0g

Hibiscus Tea

Hibiscus tea is said to keep high cholesterol and high blood pressure at bay.

Preparation time: 10 minutes
Yield: 2 servings

Ingredients
- Hibiscus Flowers (4 tbsp.)
- Water (2 cups)

Directions
1. Set your water on to boil. Once boiling add in your hibiscus and remove from heat.
2. Cover and let rest for at least 5 minutes.
3. Strain, serve and enjoy

Macros per Serving & Nutrition Facts
- Calories 9
- Total Fat 0.7 g
- Carbohydrate 0 g
- Protein 0.4 g

Green Tea

Green tea carries a myriad of health benefits, including fat loss, improving brain function, and even lowering the risk of cancer.

Preparation time: 20 minutes
Yield: 2 servings

Ingredients
- Camellia Sinensis Leaves (4 tbsp., fresh)
- Water (2 cups)

Directions

1. Set your water on to boil. Once boiling add in your Camellia and remove from heat.
2. Cover and let rest for at least 10 minutes.
3. Strain, serve and enjoy

Macros per Serving & Nutrition Facts
- Calories 10
- Total Fat 0.1 g
- Saturated Fat 0.0 g
- Carbohydrate 0 g
- Protein 0 g

Sugar Free Popsicles & Ice Treat

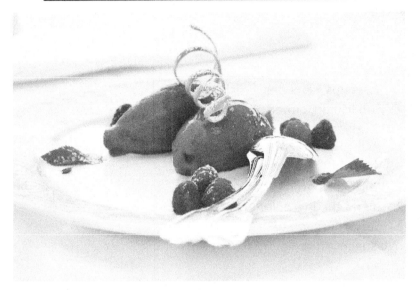

Watermelon sorbet

Watermelon sorbet tastes refreshing on the pallet.

Serves: 6
Time: 5 minutes

Ingredients:
- 4 ½ cups ice cubes, crushed
- ½lb Melon, cubed
- 1 tablespoon grated orange zest

Directions:
1. Place all ingredients in a blender.
2. Blend the ingredients for 30 seconds.
3. Serve immediately.

NB: We suggest that you make the sorbet in batches.

Macros per Serving & Nutrition Facts
- Calories 231.1
- Total Fat 0.2 g
- Carbohydrate 59.6 g
- Protein 0.6 g

Banana Icy Pops

This recipe is great for in the morning when you need a pick me up.

Serving Size: 8
Overall time: 4 hours and 30 minutes

Ingredients:
- Boiling water (1 cup)
- Fruit-flavored Jell-O (1 package)
- Banana (1)
- Plain yogurt (1 cup)

Directions:
1. Add all the ingredients in a blender. Blend everything thing until it is smooth.
2. Put mixture into a popsicle mold or an in a plastic cup.
3. Place in a freezer until hard.
4. Serve and enjoy!

Macros per Serving & Nutrition Facts
- Calories 93
- Total Fat 0.4 g
- Carbohydrate 22 g
- Protein 2.2g

Kiwi Sorbet

Cool your digestive tract with this delicious sugar free sorbet.

Serves: 6
Time: 5 minutes

Ingredients:
- 4 ½ cups ice cubes, crushed
- ½lb Kiwi, chopped
- 1 tablespoon grated orange zest

Directions:
1. Place all ingredients in a blender.
2. Blend the ingredients for 30 seconds.
3. Serve immediately.
NB: We suggest that you make the sorbet in batches.

Macros per Serving & Nutrition Facts
- Calories 105.5
- Total Fat 0.3 g
- Saturated Fat 0.0 g
- Carbohydrate 26.7 g
- Protein 0.6 g

Raspberry Icy Pops

If you love raspberry, then give these sugar free popsicles a go.

Serving Size: 8
Overall time: 4 hours and 30 minutes

Ingredients:
- Boiling water (1 cup)
- Jell-O (1 package, raspberry)
- Raspberries (1 cup, fresh)
- Plain yogurt (1 cup)

Directions:
1. Add all the ingredients in a blender. Blend everything thing until it is smooth.
2. Put mixture into a popsicle mold and place to freeze until frozen.
3. Serve and enjoy!

Macros per Serving & Nutrition Facts
- Calories 1.3
- Total Fat 0.0 g
- Carbohydrate 0.4 g
- Protein 0.0 g

Strawberry Icy Pops

These popsicles are naturally sweet and acts as a good treat in stage 1 recovery.

Serving Size: 8
Overall time: 4 hours and 30 minutes

Ingredients:
- Boiling water (1 cup)

- Fruit-flavored Jell-O (1 package)
- Strawberries (1 cup)
- Plain yogurt (1 cup)

Directions:
1. Add all the ingredients in a blender. Blend everything thing until it is smooth.
2. Put mixture into a popsicle mold or an in a plastic cup.
3. Place in a freezer until hard.
4. Serve and enjoy!

Macros per Serving & Nutrition Facts
- Calories 90
- Total Fat 1.42 g
- Carbohydrate 18.49 g
- Protein 0.71 g

Fruit Infused Water

Lemon, Mint & Cucumber Infused Water

This mix is perfect for flushing our bodies of unwanted toxins. As an added bonus, the lemons in this recipe aids in digestion while the cucumber helps to keep you refreshed and hydrated.

Makes: 48 fl. oz.
Time: 5 minutes + chilling time

Ingredients:
- 6 cups water
- 1 grapefruit, sliced
- 1 orange, sliced
- ½ cup cucumber slices

Directions
1. Combine all the ingredients in a pitcher.
2. Refrigerate for 2 hours or overnight.
3. Serve in the morning and drink through the day.

Macros per Serving & Nutrition Facts
- Calories 1.3
- Total Fat 0.0 g
- Carbohydrate 0.4 g
- Protein 0.0 g

Citrus & Mint Infused Water

Tasty and refreshing infused water that helps to promote weight loss.
Makes: 64 Fl.oz.
Time: 5 minutes + chilling time

Ingredients:
- ½ red grapefruit, segmented
- 2 mint leaves

- ½ lemon, sliced
- 1 cucumber, sliced
- ½ lime sliced
- ½ gallon spring water

Directions
1. Wash and prepare the ingredients.
2. Place all the ingredients in a pitcher.
3. Refrigerate for 2 hours.
4. Serve after.

Macros per Serving & Nutrition Facts
- Calories 2
- Total Fat 0.0 g
- Carbohydrate 0.4 g
- Protein 0.0 g

Pineapple and Mango Water

This juice will help you to boost your stamina.

Makes: 64 Fl.oz.
Time: 5 minutes + chilling time

Ingredients
- 1 cup pineapple slices
- 1 cup ripe mango, chunks
- 10 cups water
- ½ teaspoon protein powder
- 1-inch ginger sliced, peeled

Directions
1. Transfer all ingredients into a pitcher and place to chill for at least an hour.
2. Pour into serving glasses and serve.

Macros per Serving & Nutrition Facts
- Calories 10
- Total Fat 0.0 g
- Carbohydrate 12 g
- Protein 0.0 g

Honeydew & Kiwi Infused Water

If you love tropical fruits, this may just be the mix for you.

Makes: 64 Fl.oz.
Time: 5 minutes + chilling time

Ingredients:
- 1 kiwi, peeled and sliced
- 2 cups honeydew melon, chopped
- 10 cups Water

Directions
1. In a pitcher combine the fruits.
2. Fill to the top with water.
3. Refrigerate for 1 hour before serving.

Macros per Serving & Nutrition Facts
- Calories 12
- Total Fat 0.0 g
- Carbohydrate 4.4 g
- Protein 0.0 g

Sweet and Sour Lychee Infused Water

This is a unique recipe, make it and enjoy with your family members.

Makes: 64 Fl.oz.
Time: 5 minutes + chilling time

Ingredients
- 1 cup lychees, peeled, seeded
- 1 tbsp. ginger powder
- 10 cups water
- 3 tablespoons lemon juice

Directions
1. Combine all your ingredients in a pitcher.
2. Refrigerate for 1 hour before serving.

Macros per Serving & Nutrition Facts
- Calories 2
- Total Fat 0.0 g
- Carbohydrate 31g
- Protein 0.0 g

Kiwi and Kale Detox Water

Rich with calcium and omega-3 antioxidant.

Makes: 64 Fl.oz.
Time: 5 minutes + chilling time

Ingredients
- 4 kiwis, sliced
- 5 kale leaves
- 10 cups cold water

Directions
1. Combine all your ingredients in a pitcher.
2. Refrigerate for 1 hour before serving.

Macros per Serving & Nutrition Facts
- Calories 1.7
- Total Fat 0.0g
- Carbohydrate 8 g
- Protein 17 g

Honeydew & Kiwi Infused Water

If you love tropical fruits, this may just be the mix for you.

Makes: 64 fl.oz.
Time: 5 minutes + chilling time

Ingredients:
- 1 kiwi, peeled and sliced
- 2 cups honeydew melon, chopped
- 10 cups Water

Directions
1. In a pitcher combine the fruits.
2. Fill to the top with water.
3. Refrigerate for 1 hour before serving.

Macros per Serving & Nutrition Facts
- Calories 1.3
- Total Fat 0.0 g
- Carbohydrate 0.4 g
- Protein 0.0 g

Watermelon and Lemon Water

Drink this juice to prevent the diseases like asthma, clogging and airway.

Preparation time: 10 minutes
Yield: 2 servings

Ingredients
- 3 cups watermelon, chunks, seeded
- 3 tablespoons lemon juice
- 2-3 mint leaves
- 1 pinch salt

- 10 cups water

Directions
1. Combine all your ingredients in a pitcher.
2. Refrigerate for 1 hour before serving.

Macros per Serving & Nutrition Facts
- Calories 105.1
- Total Fat 1.4 g
- Carbohydrate 24.6 g
- Protein 2.1 g

Mango & Ginger Infused Water

Another refreshing drink that boosts the metabolism and promotes weight loss

Makes: 64 fl.oz.
Time: 5 minutes + chilling time

Ingredients:
- 1 cup diced mango
- 1-inch ginger, peeled and sliced
- 2 cups ice
- Water, to top off

Directions
1. Peel and slice the ginger in 3-4 coin size slices.
2. Transfer the ginger into a pitcher along with mango.
3. Top with 2 cups ice and fill with water.
4. Refrigerate for 3 hours.
5. Serve after.

Macros per Serving & Nutrition Facts
- Calories 1.3
- Total Fat 0.0 g
- Carbohydrate 0.4 g
- Protein 0.0 g

Lavender & Blueberry Infused Water

Refreshing, healthy and delicious!

Makes: 64 fl. oz.
Time: 5 minutes + chilling time

Ingredients:
- 8 cups water
- 1-pint fresh blueberries
- 1 tablespoon lavender flowers

Directions
1. Mix all your ingredients in a large pitcher.
2. Stir gently and refrigerate for 1 hour.
3. Strain and serve with ice.

Macros per Serving & Nutrition Facts
- Calories 1.3
- Total Fat 0.0 g
- Carbohydrate 0.4 g
- Protein 0.0 g

Grapefruit, Orange & Cucumber Infused Water

This mix is perfect for flushing our bodies of unwanted toxins.

Makes: 48 fl. oz.
Time: 5 minutes + chilling time

Ingredients:
- 6 cups water
- 1 grapefruit, sliced
- 1 orange, sliced
- ½ cup cucumber slices

Directions
1. Combine all the ingredients in a pitcher.
2. Refrigerate for 2 hours or overnight.
3. Serve in the morning and drink through the day.

Macros per Serving & Nutrition Facts
- Calories 1.3
- Total Fat 0.0 g
- Carbohydrate 0.4 g
- Protein 0.0 g

Pina Colada Infused Water

This recipe offers a play on the flavors of Pina Colada while maintaining a variety of health benefits.

Makes: 48 fl. oz.
Time: 5 minutes + chilling time

Ingredients:
- 1 cup peeled and thinly sliced pineapple
- 2 cups ice
- 6 cups Coconut Water

Directions
1. Pour out your pineapple into a large pitcher.
2. Top with ice.
3. Pour in water to the top and cover.
4. Refrigerate for 1 hour before serving.

Macros per Serving & Nutrition Facts
- Calories 1.3
- Total Fat 0.0 g
- Carbohydrate 0.4 g
- Protein 0.0 g

Orange & Blueberry Infused Water

A tasty blend that does well for detoxing.

Makes: 48 fl.oz.
Time: 5 minutes + chilling time

Ingredients:
- 2 oranges, cut into wedges
- 1 cup blueberries
- 6 cups water

Directions
1. Combine all ingredients in a pitcher.
2. Cover and allow to chill for a minimum of 2 hours or overnight.
3. Serve after.

Macros per Serving & Nutrition Facts
- Calories 1.3
- Total Fat 0.0 g
- Carbohydrate 0.4 g
- Protein 0.0 g

Coconut and Blueberry Infused Water

This delicious blueberry juice with coconut water is most suitable for summer.

Makes: 64 Fl.oz.
Time: 5 minutes + chilling time

Ingredients
- 3 cup blueberries
- 10 cups coconut water

Directions
1. Combine all ingredients in a pitcher.
2. Cover and allow to chill for a minimum of 2 hours or overnight.
3. Serve after.

Macros per Serving & Nutrition Facts
- Calories 9
- Total Fat 1.42 g
- Carbohydrate 8.49 g
- Protein 0.71 g

Raspberry & Orange Infused Water

This recipe offers the sweetness of the raspberries and the tanginess of the oranges; together it is simply delicious.

Makes: 48fl. oz.
Time: 5 minutes + chilling time

Ingredients:
- 2 mandarin oranges, cut into wedges
- ½ cup raspberries
- 6 cups water

Directions
1. Place all the ingredients into a pitcher.
2. Cover and allow to chill for a minimum of 2 hours or overnight.
3. Serve after.

Macros per Serving & Nutrition Facts
- Calories 1.3
- Total Fat 0.0 g
- Carbohydrate 0.4 g

Strawberry, Lemon & Basil Infused Water

This mix has become very popular in spas over the years because it promotes healthy skin, detox and even helps in boosting the metabolism.

Makes: 32 fl.oz.
Time: 5 minutes + chilling time

Ingredients:
- 6 strawberries, hulled and sliced
- ½ lemon, sliced
- 1 small handful basil, scrunched
- 4 cups water

Directions
1. In a pitcher combine all ingredients.
2. Cover and allow to chill for a minimum of 2 hours or overnight.
3. Serve after or drink through the day.

Macros per Serving & Nutrition Facts
- Calories 1.3
- Total Fat 0.0 g
- Carbohydrate 0.4 g
- Protein 0.0 g

Ginger Greens Infused Water

Vegetable water is often swallow, but this recipe aims to correct that by providing the perfect blend of vegetables and ginger.

Makes: 64 fl. Oz.
Time: 5 minutes + chilling time

Ingredients

- Water (10 cups)
- Cucumber (1 large, chopped)
- Celery (1 ½ Stalks quartered)
- Apples (2 large, seeded, quartered)
- Kale Leaves (2 Cups)
- Ginger (1-inch piece, peeled)

Directions
1. In a pitcher, combine all the ingredients.
2. Stir gently and refrigerate for at least 3 hours.
3. Serve after.

Macros per Serving & Nutrition Facts
- Calories 90.3
- Total Fat 0.0 g
- Carbohydrate 0.4 g

Carrot and Papaya Coconut Water

This is very effective for eyes health and immune system.

Makes: 64 Fl.oz.
Time: 5 minutes + chilling time

Ingredients
- 2 carrots, peeled, sliced
- 1 cup ripe papaya, chunks
- 10 cups coconut water

Directions
1. Combine all ingredients in a pitcher.
2. Cover and allow to chill for a minimum of 2 hours or overnight.
3. Serve after.

Macros per Serving & Nutrition Facts
- Calories 93
- Total Fat 0.4 g
- Carbohydrate 22 g
- Protein 2.2g

Orange, Strawberry & Mint Infused Water

If you frequently drink Mojitos, you will quickly find that replacing some of them with this mix will do wonders for your health.

Makes: 48fl. oz.
Time: 5 minutes + chilling time

Ingredients:
- 2 oranges, cut into wedges
- ½ cup strawberries
- 4 leaves mint
- 6 cups water

Directions
1. Place all the ingredients into a pitcher.
2. Cover and allow to chill for a minimum of 2 hours or overnight.
3. Serve after.

Macros per Serving & Nutrition Facts
- Calories 1.3
- Total Fat 0.0 g
- Carbohydrate 0.4 g
- Protein 0.0 g

Watermelon Infused Coconut Water

This mix is said to aid in cardiovascular health as well as rejuvenating the skin.

Makes: 32 fl.oz.
Time: 5 minutes + chilling time

Ingredients:
- 4 cups coconut water
- 4 cups watermelon
- 2 tablespoons lime juice

Directions
1. Place all ingredients in a large pitcher,
2. Muddle gently and refrigerate for 2 hours.
3. Serve after, with some ice.

Macros per Serving & Nutrition Facts
- Calories 1.3
- Total Fat 0.0 g
- Carbohydrate 0.4 g
- Protein 0.0 g

Raspberry, Kiwi & Peach Infused Water

This mix is perfect for flushing our bodies of unwanted toxins.

Makes: 64 fl. oz.
Time: 5 minutes + chilling time

Ingredients:
- 6 cups water
- 2 cups peaches, sliced
- 1 cup kiwi, sliced
- ½ cup raspberry

Directions
1. Combine all the ingredients in a pitcher.
2. Refrigerate for 2 hours or overnight.
3. Serve chilled!

Macros per Serving & Nutrition Facts
- Calories 1.3
- Total Fat 0.0 g
- Carbohydrate 0.4 g
- Protein 0.0 g

Peach & Sage Infused Water

This mix is said to provide your body with some of the required antioxidants that will help your body fight bacteria and improve your overall health.

Makes: 64 fl. oz.
Time: 5 minutes + chilling time

Ingredients:
- 1 peach, pitted and sliced
- 8 pitted and quartered plums
- 4 sage leaves, scrunched
- 8 cups water

Directions
1. In a pitcher combine all the ingredients.
2. Give it a gentle stir and refrigerate at least 2 hours.
3. Serve with ice.

Macros per Serving & Nutrition Facts
- Calories 1.3
- Total Fat 0.0 g
- Carbohydrate 0.4 g
- Protein 0.0 g

Kale & Apple Water

Though it may sound weird, this interesting blend creates a delicious and healthy juice.

Yields: 3 ½ Cups
Time Needed: 15 minutes

Ingredients
- Water (10 cups)
- Apples (4 large, seeded, quartered)
- Kale Leaves (3 Cups)
- Ginger (1-inch piece, peeled)

Directions
1. Place all the ingredients into a pitcher.
2. Cover and allow to chill for a minimum of 2 hours or overnight.
3. Serve after.

Macros per Serving & Nutrition Facts
- Calories 198
- Total Fat 3 g
- Carbohydrate 53 g
- Protein 19 g

Watermelon & Mint Infused Water

Keep your body hydrated with this refreshing cup of water.

Makes: 64 fl. oz.
Time: 5 minutes + chilling time

Ingredients:
- 2 cups diced watermelon
- 4 mint leaves

- 10 cups water

Directions
1. In a pitcher combine the grapes and oranges.
2. Muddle gently and pour in the water.
3. Refrigerate for 2 hours.
4. Serve with ice.

Macros per Serving & Nutrition Facts
- Calories 1.3
- Total Fat 0.0 g
- Carbohydrate 0.4 g
- Protein 0.0 g

Orange & Grape Infused Water

This mix is extremely tasty, offering a tangy, sweet, and refreshing mix.

Makes: 48 fl. oz.
Time: 5 minutes + chilling time

Ingredients:
- 1 cup halved red grapes, seedless
- 2 blood oranges, sliced
- 6 cups water

Directions
1. In a pitcher combine the grapes and oranges.
2. Muddle gently and pour in the water.
3. Refrigerate for 2 hours.
4. Serve with ice.

Macros per Serving & Nutrition Facts
- Calories 1.3
- Total Fat 0.0 g
- Carbohydrate 0.4 g
- Protein 0.0 g

Apple & Cinnamon Infused Water

This delicious water blend is said to boost your metabolism naturally.

Makes: 64 fl. Oz.
Time: 5 minutes + chilling time

Ingredients:
- 2 apples, thinly sliced
- 1 cinnamon stick, preferably Ceylon cinnamon
- 8 cups water
- ½ jug of ice

Directions
1. Drop the apples in the pitcher and add the cinnamon stick.
2. Fill up with the ice up to ½ way full.
3. Top off with water and refrigerate for 1 hour.
4. Serve chilled.

Macros per Serving & Nutrition Facts
- Calories 1.3
- Total Fat 0.0 g
- Carbohydrate 0.4 g
- Protein 0.0 g

Cherry Pineapple Infused Water

Use this mix to replace the sweet juices in your diet and watch in awe as the body starts to change before your eyes.

Makes: 64fl. oz.
Time: 5 minutes + chilling time

Ingredients:
- 1 cup pitted and halved cherries
- 1 cup pineapple chunks
- ½ green apple, cored and sliced
- 8 cups water

Directions
1. In a pitcher, combine all the ingredients.
2. Stir gently and refrigerate for at least 3 hours.
3. Serve after.

Macros per Serving & Nutrition Facts
- Calories 1.3
- Total Fat 0.0 g
- Carbohydrate 0.4 g
- Protein 0.0 g

Ginger Zest Beetroot Water

This glass of infused water will make your skin and hair more glowing and shinier.

Makes: 48 fl. oz.
Time: 5 minutes + chilling time

Ingredients:
- 1 cup beetroots, peeled, chunks
- 1-inch ginger sliced, peeled

- 10 cups water

Directions
1. Place all ingredients in a large pitcher,
2. Muddle gently and refrigerate for 2 hours.
3. Serve after, with some ice.

Macros per Serving & Nutrition Facts
- Calories 155
- Total Fat 1 g
- Carbohydrate 33g
- Protein 1g

Kiwi & Blackberry Infused Water

This mix is perfect for early mornings as it helps to set your metabolism in gear for the day ahead.

Makes: 32 fl. oz.
Time: 5 minutes + chilling time

Ingredients:
- ½ cup blackberries washed
- 1 kiwi, peeled and sliced
- 2 mint leaves
- 4 cups water

Directions
1. In a pitcher, combine all the ingredients.
2. Give it a gentle stir and refrigerate for 2 hours.
3. Serve after, with some ice.

Macros per Serving & Nutrition Facts
- Calories 1.3
- Total Fat 0.0 g
- Carbohydrate 0.4 g
- Protein 0.0 g

Broth Recipes

Chicken Bone Broth

This recipe is perfect for soothing stomach aches

Preparation time: 2 hours
Yield: 5 servings

Ingredients
- 1 oz. chicken bones, cleaned
- 2 tablespoons apple cider vinegar
- 1 onion, sliced
- 5-6 garlic cloves
- 1 tablespoon cooking oil
- ½ teaspoon salt
- ½ teaspoon white pepper
- 1-inch ginger slice
- 6 cups water

Directions
1. In a large skillet add bones with water, onion, garlic, ginger, oil, vinegar, salt, pepper, and stir. Cover with lid.
2. Leave to cook on low heat for 2 hours.
3. Strain the broth and discard residue.
4. Serve hot and enjoy.

Macros per Serving & Nutrition Facts
- Calories 147
- Total Fat 5 g
- Carbohydrate 9 g
- Protein 10 g

Pork Bone Broth

This highly nutritious delight is made with just a few and simple ingredients.

Preparation time: 2 hours
Yield: 5 servings

Ingredients
- 1 oz. pork bones, cleaned
- 2 tablespoons apple cider vinegar
- 1 onion, sliced
- 5-6 garlic cloves
- 1 tablespoon cooking oil
- ½ teaspoon salt
- ½ teaspoon white pepper
- 1-inch ginger slice
- 6 cups water

Directions
1. In a large skillet add bones with water, onion, garlic, ginger, oil, vinegar, salt, pepper, and stir. Cover with lid.
2. Leave to cook on low heat for 2 hours.
3. Strain the broth and discard residue.
4. Serve hot and enjoy.

Macros per Serving & Nutrition Facts
- Calories 37.7
- Total Fat 0.2 g
- Carbohydrate 8.2 g
- Protein 1 g

Conclusion

There you have it! Together we have explored 50 Amazingly Simple Recipes that you can enjoy within Stage 1 of recovery from a Gastric Sleeve Operation. We hope you will consider joining us again when we explore the remaining three stages of post operation diet procedures. Achieving a speedy and successful recovery is vital right now, and we want to help you get there. See you next time.

Gastric Sleeve Cookbook Stage 2

50 Delicious Protein Shakes & Smoothies, Soups and Puddings Recipes You Can Enjoy in Stage 2 Post Weight Loss Surgery Rehabilitation

Table of Contents

Introduction

Congratulations, once again, on successfully completing your gastric sleeve surgery and making it successfully into your second stage of the recovery diet! So, stage 1 consuming only clear fluids was a success, and you are ready to move on to stage 2 which primarily has thicker liquids and slowly introducing smooth foods into the diet. Before you proceed to this stage it is important that you check your fluid consumption log and ask yourself if you can comfortably consume a suitable amount of liquid daily without experiencing added pouch irritation, discomfort, and vomiting? If so, then great; feel free to move on to stage 2 confidently. However, if you are still not quite there, don't rush yourself. Instead, consider sticking to stage 1 for a few more days to a week until you are able to comfortably move on. Remember, every patient is different so your body may heal differently than others. Listen to your body, and adjust your recovery process to suit your body and specific needs.

So, what should you expect to achieve in Stage 2?

In this stage of your diet you will be introducing more full liquids to your diet, so when you are just transitioning from stage 1, you will start to try your body with digesting more shakes, milk, skimmed milk, sugar free soft puddings, and maybe even sugar free porridges. In this stage, you want to aim to consume at least 6 to 8 fluid ounces of liquid per hour while taking more frequent smaller portions of food. Then towards the end of the stage when you begin to transition to stage 3 then you will start testing yourself with the introduction of soft or smooth foods in an attempt to get your body prepared for stage 3. Don't be scared! You can definitely get through this. Just ensure that you keep these few key tips in mind as you go through this stage.

Stage 2 Key Tips/Reminders

- In this stage protein shakes will be your best friend. Meeting your nutritional targets daily as the stages go by will become more and more vital to a tall glass of a protein shake will help you along with meeting those pesky protein targets.
- When you get into the second week of this stage when you begin to introduce smooth foods to your diet, be sure that you do not force yourself to eat. Listen to your body! If you do not feel really hungry, opt to try drinking a small glass of protein shake versus a whole serving of your scheduled smooth meal.
- Be sure that you pace yourself while you eat. Try to take dime sized bites and allow your body to process that before jumping to binge on more.
- When you begin to try smooth foods, aim to have your food the consistency of apple sauce so that it can be easily digested without too much discomfort. Even if your food appears to be smooth always chew thoroughly before attempting to swallow.
- It is important to stay hydrated! Try to continue t sip on clear fluids in between meals. Try not to drink too much close to your schedule meal times as you want to leave space in your stomach for the actual meal. Remember your stomach is not able to hold as much as it could before so over eating may result in vomiting or discomfort.
- Keep a log of the nutrients you are consuming and be sure to supplement the nutrients you fall short on (many patients fall short on their protein, B12, and Calcium intake during the first couple of stages so check with your doctor if taking a pill is necessary in your case).
- Try to eat at set times throughout the day and stick to it. That way you can ensure you are actually consuming enough food for your body. Try to eat at least every 4 hours while you are awake.
- Aim to consume at least 64 fluid ounces of liquid each day. This may sound like a lot, however, remember that there is

liquid in your shakes so track that first then supplement your fluid intake with clear liquids throughout the day.

This is a lot of information to take in, but it really isn't as complicated as it sounds. In this Gastric Sleeve Cookbook, we are going to help keep you on track with 50 Delicious recipe suggestions that you can enjoy in Stage 2 of your post gastric sleeve recovery diet. We guarantee that once you see how simple it can be things will begin to become clearer. So, without further ado, let's get started.

Introducing Full Liquids

Protein Shakes & Smoothies

Pineapple Shake V 20

This sweet and tasty drink is a brilliant end to a heavy meal.

Serves: 6
Time: 20 minutes

Ingredients:
- Frozen pineapple (3 cups)
- Whey Protein Powder (2 scoops)
- Greek yogurt (1 cup, pineapple/vanilla flavored)
- Unsweetened vanilla almond milk (1 cup)
- Vanilla extract (1 tbs.)

Directions:
1. Add the ingredients in the blender and blend until smooth.
2. Serve and enjoy!

Macros per Serving & Nutrition Facts
- Calories 580
- Total Fat 31 g
- Total Carbohydrate 68 g
- Protein 28g

Blueberry Cacao Blast V 20

Simple yet delicious dessert smoothie.

Serves: 1
Time: 5 minutes

Ingredients:
- 1 cup blueberries
- 1 tablespoon raw cacao nibs
- 1 tablespoon Chia seeds
- 1 dash cinnamon

- ½ Spinach (chopped)
- ½ Cup Bananas (chopped)
- 1½ Cup Almond milk
- 2 scoops Whey protein powder

Directions:
1. Place raspberries, cacao nibs, Chia seeds and cinnamon in a blender.
2. Add enough almond milk to reach the max line.
3. Process for 30 seconds or until you get a smooth mixture.
4. Serve immediately in the chilled tall glass.

Macros per Serving & Nutrition Facts
- Calories 321
- Total Fat 2.7 g
- Total Carbohydrate 69.4 g
- Protein 24.7g

Cucumber and Avocado Dill Smoothie V 20

If you are looking for a delicious and healthy smoothie, then this is perfect for you.

Serves: 2
Time: 5 minutes

Ingredients:
- 1 cucumber, peeled, sliced
- 2 tablespoons dill, chopped
- 2 tablespoons lemon juice
- 1 avocado, pitted
- 1 cup coconut milk
- 1 teaspoon coconut, shredded
- 2 kiwis, peeled, sliced

Directions
1. In a blender add all ingredients and blend well.
2. Drain the extract and discard residue.
3. Serve and enjoy.

Macros per Serving & Nutrition Facts
- Calories 165
- Total Fat 5.5 g
- Total Carbohydrate 24.8 g
- Protein 2.3g

Spinach Green Smoothie V 20

This smoothie will definitely blow your mind by its taste and freshness.

Serves: 2
Time: 5 min

Ingredients:
- 1 cup baby spinach leaves
- 2-3 mint leave
- 1 cup 100% grapes juice
- 1 cup 100% pineapple juice
- 2 tablespoons lime juice
- 2 scoops protein powder

Directions
1. In a blender add ingredients and blend well till puree.
2. Transfer to serving glasses.
3. Serve and enjoy.

Macros per Serving & Nutrition Facts
- Calories 268
- Total Fat 5.5 g
- Total Carbohydrate 11.4 g
- Protein 24.3g

Coco - Banana Milkshake V 20

Here is a delicious milkshake that is naturally sweet from the coconut and bananas.

Serves: 1
Time: 5 minutes

Ingredients
- 1 cup coconut milk
- 2 ripe bananas
- 2 tablespoons cinnamon
- ¼ teaspoon cardamom powder
- 2 scoops protein powder
- 7 ice cubes

Directions
1. In a blender add coconut milk with cardamom powder, cinnamon, bananas and blend well.
2. Pour into glass and add ice chunks.
3. Serve and enjoy.

Macros per Serving & Nutrition Facts
- Calories 191.9
- Total Fat 7.1g
- Total Carbohydrate 35.8 g
- Protein 25.7g

Strawberry and Cherry Shake V 20

This shake is absolutely a great boost with wonderful taste.

Serves:2
Time: 5 minutes

Ingredients:

- 1 cup strawberries
- 1 cup cherries
- 1 cup almond milk
- ½ cup coconut milk
- 2 scoops protein powder
- Few ice chunks

Directions
1. In a blender add all ingredients and blend well.
2. Serve and enjoy.

Macros per Serving & Nutrition Facts
- Calories 138
- Total Fat 0g
- Total Carbohydrate 30 g
- Protein 20g

Chia Blueberry Banana Oatmeal Smoothie V 20

Banana check, blueberry check, starting the day right, check.

Serves: 1
Time: 10m

Ingredients:
- Soy milk (1 cups)
- Frozen banana (1, sliced)
- Frozen blueberries (1/4 cup)
- Oats (1/4 cup)
- Vanilla extract (1 tsp.)
- Cinnamon (1 tsp., to taste)
- Chia seed (1 tbs.)

Directions:
1. Add all ingredients into a blender and blend until the ingredients are combined and smooth.

2. Serve and enjoy!

Macros per Serving & Nutrition Facts
- Calories 178
- Total Fat 4.2 g
- Total Carbohydrate 36.2 g
- Protein 3.2 g

Chocolate Coconut Chia Smoothie V 20

This smoothie is packed with protein and filled with sweet chocolaty flavor.

Serves: 1
Time: 5 minutes

Ingredients:
- 1 tablespoon raw cacao nibs
- 1 tablespoon Chia seeds
- 1 dash cinnamon
- ½ Spinach (chopped)
- ½ Cup Coconut (shredded)
- 1½ Cup Almond milk

Directions:
1. Place coconut, cacao nibs, Chia seeds and cinnamon in Vitamix.
2. Add enough almond milk to reach the max line.
3. Process for 30 seconds or until you get a smooth mixture.
4. Serve immediately in the tall chilled glass.

Macros per Serving & Nutrition Facts
- Calories 480
- Total Fat 22 g
- Total Carbohydrate 55 g
- Protein 30 g

Banana-Cherry Smoothie V 20

Cherries are great in combatting inflammation in the body and

Serves: 1
Time: 5 minutes

Ingredients:
- 1 banana
- 1 cup cherries, pitted
- ¼ teaspoon nutmeg
- 1scoop protein powder
- 1 cup almond milk

Directions:
1. Place all ingredients in a blender
2. Process ingredients until smooth, for 20 seconds.
3. Serve immediately.

Macros per Serving & Nutrition Facts
- Calories 398
- Total Fat 2 g
- Total Carbohydrate 89.2 g
- Protein 17 g

Avocado Smoothie V 20

This recipe produces a creamy and delicious green smoothie providing a healthy source of fat.

Serves: 1
Time: 5 minutes

Ingredients:
- 1 medium ripe avocado
- ¼ cup crushed peanuts
- 1 tablespoon flax seed
- 1 ½ cups vanilla Greek yogurt
- 1 cup Liquid (milk, water, coconut milk, etc.)

Directions:
1. Place all ingredients in Vitamix.
2. Process ingredients until smooth, for 20 seconds.
3. Serve immediately.

Macros per Serving & Nutrition Facts
- Calories 592
- Total Fat 22 g
- Total Carbohydrate 96 g
- Protein 3 g

Mango Smoothie V 20

Enjoy this rich tropical mango smoothie that will remind you of the islands.

Serves: 2
Time: 5 minutes

Ingredients:
- 2 Mangos (seeded, diced, frozen)
- Milk (1 cup)
- ½ cup crushed ice
- 1 cup plain yogurt
- 2 scoops protein powder

Directions:
1. Combine all ingredients in Vitamix.
2. Process for 30 seconds or until smooth.
3. Serve immediately in a tall glass.

Macros per Serving & Nutrition Facts
- Calories 320
- Total Fat 0 g
- Total Carbohydrate 78 g
- Protein 21 g

Homemade Unsweetened Milk

Cashew Milk V 20

Who says you have to pay a fortune for Cashew Milk? Get fresh homemade cashew milk using your Vitamix right from your kitchen.

Serves: 5
Time:15min.

Ingredients
- Cashew (1 Cup. Soaked over time)
- Water (4 cups)
- Dates (3)

DIRECTIONS
1. Add all your ingredients to your Vitamix.
2. Pulse for until creamy (should take about 1 min).
3. Enjoy!

Macros per Serving & Nutrition Facts
- Calories 60
- Total Fat 2.5 g
- Total Carbohydrate 27.3 g
- Protein 8 g

Almond Milk V 20

Almond milk does not have to be expensive. Using this recipe, you can enjoy fresh Almond Milk from your kitchen.

Serves: 5 cups
Time Needed: 15min.

Ingredients
- Almonds (1 Cup. Soaked over time)
- Water (4 cups)

Directions
1. Add all your ingredients to your Vitamix.
2. Pulse for until creamy (should take about 1 min).
3. Enjoy!

Macros per Serving & Nutrition Facts
- Calories 90
- Total Fat 2.5 g
- Total Carbohydrate 16 g
- Protein 1 g

Strained Soups

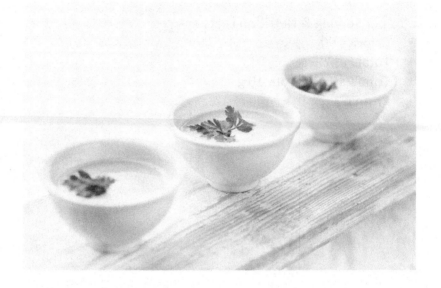

Pumpkin and carrot soup V 20

Super healthy and vibrant soup everyone will love.

Serves: 4
Time: 20 minutes

Ingredients:
- 0.5 lb. pumpkin puree
- 0.5 lb. carrots, cut into ½-inch pieces
- 2 cups vegetable stock
- ½ cup chopped onion
- Fresh ground salt and pepper – to taste
- 1 teaspoon dried thyme
- 2 oz. cauliflower florets
- ½ tablespoon olive oil
- 1 anise star

Direction:
1. Heat olive oil in medium pot and add onion; add cauliflower, carrots and sauté for 15 minutes, until onion is caramelized.
2. Add thyme and stir well.
3. Transfer the vegetables in a Nutri Bullet, add pumpkin puree, vegetable stock, and pulse until smooth.
4. Transfer the mixture into sauce pan and simmer, add anise star and simmer over medium-high heat for 5-8 minutes or until heated through.
5. Remove the anise star and discard.
6. Strain through a fine sieve or cheesecloth and serve immediately.

Macros per Serving & Nutrition Facts
- Calories 70
- Total Fat 0 g
- Total Carbohydrate 0 g
- Protein 2 g

Super Soup

Why Super soup? Well, it is packed with the super ingredients and has a super taste.

Serves: 6
Time: 30 minutes

Ingredients:
- 14oz. cauliflower heat, cut into florets
- 5oz. watercress
- 7oz. spinach, thawed
- 4 cups chicken stock
- 1 cup coconut milk
- ¼ cup ghee
- Salt and pepper – to taste
- 1 onion, chopped
- 2 garlic cloves, crushed

Directions:
1. Grease Dutch oven with ghee, place over medium-high heat and add onion and garlic. Cook until browned and stir cauliflower florets. Cook for 5 minutes.
2. Add spinach and water cress and cook for 2 minutes or until just wilted, pour in vegetable stock and bring to boil.
3. Cook until cauliflower is crisp-tender and stir in the coconut milk.
4. Season with salt and pepper and remove from the heat. Allow cooling and puree the soup in Nutri Bullet until creamy.
5. Strain through a fine sieve or cheesecloth and serve immediately.

Macros per Serving & Nutrition Facts
- Calories 392
- Total Fat 37.6 g

- Total Carbohydrate 9.7 g
- Protein 4.9 g

Tomato bisque

This soup has a kind of pizza aroma. It is filled with tomatoes and basil.

Serves: 4
Time: 30 minutes

Ingredients:
- 28oz. tomatoes, peeled and pureed
- 1 cup coconut cream
- 1 onion, diced
- 1 teaspoon fresh ground pepper
- 4 cups chicken stock
- 1 bunch celery, chopped
- ½ cup basil, chopped
- 1 tablespoon olive oil
- Salt and pepper – to taste

Directions:
1. Heat olive oil in large pot over medium-high heat, add onion, with celery and cook until tender.
2. Pour chicken stock and tomatoes in the pot, bring mixture to simmer and season with salt and pepper. Simmer for 30 minutes.
3. Turn off heat and allow the soup to cool down. Puree in Nutri Bullet in batches.
4. Stir in heavy cream, basil, and Parmesan cheese.
5. Strain through a fine sieve or cheesecloth and serve immediately.

Macros per Serving & Nutrition Facts
- Calories 140
- Total Fat 7 g
- Total Carbohydrate 17 g
- Protein 3 g

Smoky soup V

Soup made with smoked paprika, bell peppers and with a pinch of ginger.

Serves: 4
Time: 40 minutes

Ingredients:
- 3 red bell peppers, diced
- 1 ½ tablespoons grass-fed butter
- 2 carrots, grated
- 1 brown onion, diced
- 2 garlic cloves, minced
- 1 ½ tablespoon tomato puree
- 2 teaspoons fresh grated ginger
- 1 teaspoon smoked paprika
- 1 bay leaf
- ½ cup chilled coconut cream whisked with 1 tablespoon lemon juice
- 4 cups homemade vegetable stock
- ½ teaspoon ground coriander

Directions:
1. Melt butter in medium heavy-bottom pan, over medium-high heat.
2. Add carrots, bell peppers, and onion. Cook for 13-15 minutes or until onion is golden, stirring occasionally.
3. Add garlic, ginger, smoked paprika, tomato puree and coriander.

4   Cook until very fragrant, for 2 minutes.
5   Add bay leaf and stock; bring to boil and reduce heat to medium-low and simmer for 20-25 minutes.
6   Remove bay leaf and when cooled puree in batches using Nutribullet. Process until smooth.
7   Stir Strain in a fine sieve or cheesecloth and serve immediately.

Macros per Serving & Nutrition Facts
- Calories 100
- Total Fat 2 g
- Total Carbohydrate 16 g
- Protein 5 g

Chicken Ramen Soup Broth

If you love ramen, you will love this recipe. It uses chicken instead of pork for all the chicken lovers.

Serves: 2-3
Time: 1 hr.

Ingredients:
- Onion, large, diced (1)
- Carrots, diced (2)
- Celery, diced (3)
- Garlic, finely chopped (4 cloves)
- Kosher salt (1 tsp)
- Pepper (½ tsp)
- Cinnamon (2 tsp)
- Chicken broth, low sodium (6)
- Light Miso (2 tsp)
- Chicken breasts (1 lb.)
- Spinach (1 bag)

Directions

1. Prepare carrots, celery, and onions for cooking in a latch Dutch oven for 5-7 minutes over medium heat. Now include salt, pepper, cinnamon, and garlic, and continue to cook for an additional minute.
2. Add chicken broth and miso before bringing to a boil.
3. Now add whole chicken breasts (raw), and simmer. Continue for 10-12 minutes. Occasionally remove a chicken breast and cut it, to see if it is cooked.
4. When the chicken is cooked thoroughly, relocate it to a cutting board for cooling.
5. When the chicken is cool enough to be handled, mince it finely, then add it back into the vegetable broth.
6. Stir in spinach to cook for approximately 5 minutes until spinach is tender.
7. Serve and enjoy!

Macros per Serving & Nutrition Facts
- Calories 326.9
- Total Fat 13.4 g
- Total Carbohydrate 39.7 g
- Protein 10.3 g

Carrot, Ginger Gusto Apple Soup

You will be surprised with this yummy soup.

Serves: 3
Preparation time: 35 minutes

Ingredients:
- 2 cup yellow apple, chunks, peeled
- 1 cup boiled chicken, shredded
- 1 carrot, peeled and chopped
- ¼ cup cherries, chopped

- 2 cups chicken broth
- 1 tablespoons lemon juice
- 1 teaspoon ginger paste
- ½ teaspoon black pepper
- ¼ teaspoon salt
- 1 tablespoon oil

Directions
1. Heat oil in a pan, add ginger paste and fry for 1 minute.
2. Add all chicken and carrots, then fry well.
3. Season with salt and pepper.
4. Transfer apple chunks, strawberries, chicken broth and stir well.
5. Place to cook on low fire for 30 minutes.
6. Drizzle lemon juice.
7. Strain, and ladle into serving bowls.
8. Serve and enjoy.

Macros per Serving & Nutrition Facts
- Calories 172.3
- Total Fat 8.7 g
- Total Carbohydrate 22.7 g
- Protein 3.2 g

Carrot, Ginger Zest Chicken Orangey Soup 20

This soup is the combination of orange slices and chicken with the flavor of ginger.

Serves: 3
Time: 15 minutes

Ingredients:
- 1 oz. chicken bones or boiled chicken feet
- 2 oranges, sliced, seeded

- 2 carrots, peeled and chopped
- 2 cups chicken broth
- 1 teaspoon ginger paste
- ½ teaspoon chili powder
- ¼ teaspoon salt
- 1 tablespoon oil

Directions
1. Heat oil in a pan, add ginger paste and carrot, then cook for 1 minute.
2. Add chicken, salt, chili powder and fry till golden brown.
3. Add chicken broth, orange slice and stir.
4. Leave to cook on low heat for 15 minutes.
5. Strain and ladle into serving bowls.
6. Serve and enjoy.

Macros per Serving & Nutrition Facts
- Calories 159
- Total Fat 3 g
- Total Carbohydrate 27 g
- Protein 6 g

Rice Cooker Garden soup

Enjoy delicious soup made of different veggies and chewy bulgur.

Serves: 6
Time: 50 minutes

Ingredients:
- 15oz. can chickpeas, rinsed and drained
- 2 carrots, diced
- 2 zucchinis, trimmed, cubed
- 2 sprigs thyme
- 1 leek, white and light green parts chopped
- ½ cup bulgur

- 4oz. green beans, cut into ½-inch pieces
- 6 cups water
- 2 garlic cloves, minced
- 2 cups chicken stock
- 2 tablespoons butter
- 1 cup tomatoes, chopped
- 1 cup fresh peas
- 1 bay leaf
- Salt and pepper, to taste

Directions:
1. Set your rice cooker to white rice.
2. Add the butter and once melted add the celery, chickpeas, leek, garlic, zucchinis, garlic.
3. Cook, stirring for 4 minutes.
4. Add the stock, bulgur, tomatoes, bay leaf, water, and thyme.
5. Simmer for 30 minutes. Add the green beans and peas. Discard the thyme. Cook for 5 minutes.
6. Serve after.

Macros per Serving & Nutrition Facts
- Calories 100
- Total Fat 3.5 g
- Total Carbohydrate 18 g
- Protein 3 g

Lemony Chicken Soup Broth

A zest of fresh lemon juice infuses this tasty Chicken soup. Other rich spices help to make the experience fun!

Serves: 2-3
Time: 1 hr.
Ingredients
- Onion, large, diced (1)

- Carrots, diced (2)
- Celery, diced (3)
- Garlic, finely chopped (4 cloves)
- Kosher salt (1 tsp)
- Pepper (½ tsp)
- Cinnamon (2 tsp)
- Chicken broth, low sodium (6)
- Parsley, extra for garnish (10 sprigs)
- Chicken breasts (1 lb.)
- Spinach (1 bag)
- Chick peas, canned, washed/drained (15 ounces)
- Juice of a Lemon (½ lemon, or more to taste)

Directions
1. Prepare carrots, celery, and onions for cooking in a latch Dutch oven for 5-7 minutes over medium heat. Now include salt, pepper, cinnamon, and garlic, and continue to cook for an additional minute.
2. Add whole parsley sprigs to your pot and stir in chicken broth before bringing to a boil.
3. Now add whole chicken breasts (raw), and simmer. Continue for 10-12 minutes. Occasionally remove a chicken breast and cut it, to see if it is cooked.
4. When the chicken is cooked thoroughly, relocate it to a cutting board for cooling.
5. When the chicken is cool enough to be handled, shred it, then add it back into the vegetable broth.
6. Stir in lemon juice, chick peas, and spinach to cook for approximately 5 minutes until spinach is tender.
7. Strain the soup to gather the broth and discard the solids, garnish with newly chopped parsley, and enjoy!

Macros per Serving & Nutrition Facts
- Calories 252.8
- Total Fat 8 g
- Total Carbohydrate 19.8 g
- Protein 25.6 g

Introducing Smooth & Pureed Foods

Sugar Free Puddings & Treats

Chocolate and Banana Pudding V

Make this pudding and place in the fridge for better results.

Serves: 5
Preparation time: 2 hours

Ingredients
- 1 cup almond milk
- 1 cup chocolate, melted
- 4 bananas, peeled, sliced
- ½ cup condensed almond milk
- 2 tablespoons butter
- 2 tablespoons cocoa powder
- 1 cup coconut cream

Directions
1. In a sauce pan add butter with and leave to cook until reduced to half.
2. Now add condensed almond milk, chocolate, cocoa powder, and stir gradually.
3. Pour half of chocolate pudding into a large dish and place banana slices evenly.
4. Pour remaining chocolate on top and freeze for 2 hours.
5. Top with whipped cream before serving.
6. Enjoy.

Macros per Serving & Nutrition Facts

- Calories 187.3
- Total Fat 3.6 g
- Total Carbohydrate 34.7 g
- Protein 4.4 g

Pomegranate Pudding V

This recipe is sugar free, and it has pomegranate for added sweetness

Serves: 4
Time: 4 hours and 35 minutes

Ingredients:
- Pomegranate juice (1 cup)
- Pomegranate juice (1/4 cup)
- Agar Agar flakes (1 tbs.)
- Tapioca starch (1 tsp.)
- Protein Powder (1 scoop)

Directions:
1. In a saucepan add the 1 cup of pomegranate juice and the agar agar. On medium heat bring it to a simmer and stir occasionally. Once the pot starts to simmer, lower the temperature to a lower heat for a 1 minute.
2. In a cup add the ¼ cup of the remaining pomegranate juice and the tapioca. Stir well. Add this mixture to the sauce pan and stir well.
3. Pour the mixture into a serving cup and put it in the fridge for 4 hours so that the Jell-O set.
4. Serve and enjoy!

Macros per Serving & Nutrition Facts
- Calories 57
- Total Fat 0 g
- Total Carbohydrate 12 g
- Protein 12 g

Carrot Pudding V

Creamy carrot pudding with a delicate lemony aroma.

Serves: 6
Time: 30 minutes

Ingredients:
- 2/3 cup Carrot Puree
- 1 teaspoon vanilla paste
- 1 teaspoon lemon zest
- 4 cups coconut milk
- Cornstarch Slurry (mixture of 2 tbs. cornstarch and 4tbs. water)
- 1 egg

Directions:
1. Place the carrot and milk into a saucepan over low heat.
2. Cover and cook until tiny bubbles begin to form.
3. Meanwhile, whisk the egg, cornstarch slurry, and lemon zest then add to the pot in a steady stream.
4. Cover and cook for 15 minutes.
5. Divide the mix between dessert bowls.
6. Cool before serving.

Macros per Serving & Nutrition Facts
- Calories 159
- Total Fat 10 g
- Total Carbohydrate 18 g
- Protein 4 g

Yogurt Crème Brulee Custard V 20

Who says a yogurt can be served only in one way? We bring you something really special.

Serves: 4
Time: 5 minutes

Ingredients:
- 2 cup thick Greek yogurt
- 1 cup strawberries puree

Directions:
1. In a bowl, combine the strawberries puree with yogurt.
2. Divide the mix between four ramekins.
3. Serve after.

Macros per Serving & Nutrition Facts
- Calories 357.6
- Total Fat 27 g
- Total Carbohydrate 22.2 g
- Protein 5.9 g

Mango Chia Pudding V

Now you can enjoy the taste of mango in the morning.

Serves: 6
Time: 2h 10m

Ingredients:
- Flax milk (1 ½ cups, coconut flavored)
- Large mango (1, cut into chunks)
- Vanilla extract (1 tsp.)
- Tea salt (1/8 tsp.)
- Chia seed (7 tbs.)
- Cinnamon (3 tbs.)

Directions:
1. Add all ingredients into a blender and blend until the ingredients are combined and smooth.
2. Put the mixture into a bowl and it in the fridge for 2 hours or until it thickens.

3. Serve and enjoy!

Macros per Serving & Nutrition Facts
- Calories 159
- Total Fat 10 g
- Total Carbohydrate 18 g
- Protein 4 g

Chocolate Mousse V 20

Chocolate mousse prepared in a blender. Rich and decadent.

Serves: 2
Time: 5 minutes

Ingredients:
- ¼ cup unsweetened dark chocolate
- 1¾ cups heavy whipping cream
- ½ teaspoon orange extract
- ¼ Cup cinnamon
- ½ cup whip cream (to serve)
- ¼ cup dark unsweetened chocolate (shaved, to serve)

Directions:
1. Place all ingredients into a blender.
2. Process until desired consistency is reached.
3. Chill, and top with whip cream and shaved chocolate before serving.

Macros per Serving & Nutrition Facts
- Calories 40
- Total Fat 3 g
- Total Carbohydrate 3 g
- Protein 1 g

Lemon Crème Brulee Custard V

Creamy, tasty and decadent without the super crunchy sugar crust.

Serves: 5
Time: 50 minutes + inactive time

Ingredients:
- 8 egg yolks, whisked
- 1 tablespoons cinnamon
- ½ teaspoon lemon extract
- 1 teaspoon lemon zest
- ½ teaspoon vanilla extract
- 2 cups heavy coconut cream, chilled

Directions:
1. In a large heavy-bottom sauce pan, over medium heat, heat whipping cream cinnamon until bubbly around the sides of the pan.
2. Remove from the heat and add 1 tablespoon of heated cream into egg yolks; whisk well and pour the egg mixture into hot cream, stirring constantly.
3. Stir in the extracts and lemon zest, whisking well.
4. Preheat oven to 325F and pour the mixture into six 6 oz. ramekins.
5. Place ramekins into baking pan and pour around 1 cup water; set in the oven and bake uncovered for 30 minutes or until center is just set.
6. Remove ramekins from the hot bath and cook for 10 minutes.
7. Cover and refrigerate for 4 hours.
8. Serve immediately.

Macros per Serving & Nutrition Facts
- Calories 198
- Total Fat 15.7 g

- Total Carbohydrate 12.2 g
- Protein 2.6 g

Raisin and Oats Mug Cakes V 20

Do you love oatmeal and want another way to make a creative dish with them? Why not make a mug cake?

Serves: 1
Time: 3 minutes

Ingredients
- Flour (1 ½ tbsp.)
- Almond milk (1 ½ tbsp.)
- Raisins (1/2 tbsp.)
- Baking powder (1/4 teaspoon)
- Salt (1/16 tsp. to taste)
- Canola oil (1/2 tbsp.)
- Baking soda (1/8 teaspoons)
- Vanilla extract (1/8 teaspoon)
- Hazelnut extract (1/8 teaspoon)
- Oats (3/4 tbsps., apple cinnamon)
- Lemon Juice (1 tsp.)

Directions
1 Whisk all ingredients in a microwavable mug and place to cook on high for a minute.
2 Cool, serve and enjoy!

Macros per Serving & Nutrition Facts
- Calories 185
- Total Fat 1.7 g
- Total Carbohydrate 39.9 g
- Protein 7.6 g

Thicker/Creamier Soups

Onion and Peas Soup

A simple and colorful soup that with blow your mind.

Serves: 3
Time: 25 minutes

Ingredients
- 1 cup peas, boiled
- 2 carrots, peeled, chopped
- 1 onion, sliced
- 2 cups chicken broth
- 1 tablespoons lemon juice
- 4-5 garlic cloves, minced
- ½ teaspoon black pepper
- ¼ teaspoon salt
- 1 tablespoon oil

Directions
1. Heat oil in a saucepan, add onion and garlic cloves, fry for 2 minutes.
2. Add all peas and carrots stir for 5 minutes.
3. Add chicken broth, salt, pepper, and mix well.
4. Leave to cook on low heat for 15 minutes.
5. Strain and ladle into serving bowls.
6. Drizzle lemon juice.
7. Serve and enjoy.

Macros per Serving & Nutrition Facts
- Calories 115
- Total Fat 0 g
- Total Carbohydrate 21 g
- Protein 7 g

Curried Carrot, Sweet Potato, and Ginger Soup V

Cholesterol isn't an issue when enjoying this delicious creamy soup, as it Is filled with Beta-Carotene and Vitamin A which together helps to promote healthy vision.

Serves: 3
Time: 30 – 35min

Ingredients:
- Extra Virgin Olive Oil (2 tsp.)
- Shallots (½ cup, chopped)
- Sweet Potato (3 cups, peeled, cubed)
- Carrots (1½ cup, peeled, sliced)

Directions:
1 Place a saucepan with your oil on medium heat until it just begins to smoke.
2 Add your shallots to the pot and sauté until it becomes tender (should take approximately 2 – 3 min).
3 Add all your prepped vegetables to the shallots, and your curry then allow to cook for another 2 minutes.
4 Pour in your broth and allow it to come to a boil. Once boiling, place the lid on the pot and reduce the heat to low.
5 Allow this mixture to simmer until your vegetables are all tender.
6 Once tender, add salt and pour your soup into a food processor. Pulse until creamy and smooth.
7 Strain, serve and Enjoy.

Tip: Consider topping with a teaspoon of vanilla Greek yogurt and sesame seeds.

Macros per Serving & Nutrition Facts
- Calories 144
- Total Fat 2.3 g
- Total Carbohydrate 27.3 g
- Protein 4.1 g

Creamy Cauliflower Soup

Get a creamy cauliflower soup just like they do in the restaurants.

Serves: 6
Time: 30 minutes

Ingredients:
- 14oz. cauliflower heat, cut into florets
- 5oz. watercress
- 7oz. spinach, thawed
- cups chicken stock
- ¼ cup ghee
- Salt and pepper – 1 tsp. each to taste
- 1 onion, chopped
- garlic cloves, crushed

Directions:
1. Grease Dutch oven with ghee, place over medium-high heat and add onion and garlic. Cook until browned and stir cauliflower florets. Cook for 5 minutes.
2. Add spinach and water cress and cook for 2 minutes or until just wilted, pour in vegetable stock and bring to boil.
3. Cook until cauliflower is crisp-tender and stir in the coconut milk.
4. Season with salt and pepper and remove from the heat. Allow cooling and puree the soup in Vitamix until creamy.
5. Strain and serve immediately.

Macros per Serving & Nutrition Facts
- Calories 105
- Total Fat 8 g
- Total Carbohydrate 6 g
- Protein 4 g

Cream of Corn Soup V

This classic and delicious treat can become even more smooth when finished in a Vitamix.

Serves: 4
Time Needed: 25 minutes

Ingredients:
- 0.5 lb. Corn puree
- 0.5 lb. carrots, cut into ½-inch pieces
- 2 cups vegetable stock
- ½ cup chopped onion
- ½ teaspoon Salt
- ¼ teaspoon Pepper
- 1 teaspoon dried thyme
- 2 oz. celery (chopped)
- ½ tablespoon olive oil
- 1 anise star

Directions:
1. Heat olive oil in medium pot and add onion; add celery, carrots and sauté for 15 minutes, until onion is caramelized. Add in corn and stir until corn is tender.
2. Add thyme and stir well.
3. Transfer the vegetables in a Vitamix, add pumpkin puree, vegetable stock, and pulse until smooth.
4. Transfer the mixture into sauce pan and simmer, add anise star and simmer over medium-high heat for 5-8 minutes or until heated through.
5. Remove the anise star and discard.
6. Serve immediately.

Macros per Serving & Nutrition Facts
- Calories 294
- Total Fat 8.3 g
- Total Carbohydrate 56 g
- Protein 12.9 g

Chestnut Soup

The soup is a combination of heavy cream, roasted chestnuts, and bacon. The perfect soup for the perfect autumn day.

Serves: 6
Time: 45 minutes

Ingredients:
- 30oz. whole roasted chestnuts
- 1 shallot, roughly chopped
- bacon slices, chopped
- ½ cup heavy cream
- ½ cups chicken stock
- 1 leek, white and light green parts chopped
- 2 tablespoons butter
- 1 sprig thyme
- 1 bay leaf
- 1 celery stalk, chopped
- ½ teaspoon nutmeg
- Salt and pepper, to taste

Directions:
1. Cook bacon in an in a medium saucepot for 3-4 minutes.
2. Add butter, carrot, leek, shallot, and celery. Cook for 6-7 minutes or until veggies are tender.
3. Add stock, thyme, bay leaf, chestnuts and bring to boil. Reduce heat and simmer for 25 minutes.
4. Remove from the heat and discard the thyme and bay leaf. Allow to cool slightly and puree using an immersion blender.
5. Reheat the soup and stir in the cream, nutmeg and season to taste. Cook for 5 minutes more. Serve while still hot.

Macros per Serving & Nutrition Facts
- Calories 280
- Total Fat 18 g
- Total Carbohydrate 25 g
- Protein 6 g

Coconut Mushroom Soup

This soup is made with mushrooms cooked in coconut milk.

Serves: 3
Preparation time: 25 minutes

Ingredients
- 1 cup mushrooms, sliced
- 1 cup coconut milk
- 1 onion, sliced
- 1 cup chicken broth
- 4-5 garlic cloves, minced
- ½ teaspoon black pepper
- ¼ teaspoon salt
- 1 tablespoon oil

Directions
1. Heat oil in a saucepan, add onion and garlic cloves, cook for 1 minute.
2. Add all mushroom and fry for 5 minutes.
3. Add chicken broth, coconut milk, salt, pepper and mix well.
4. Leave to cook on low heat for 15 minutes.
5. Transfer to serving bowls.
6. Serve and enjoy.

Macros per Serving & Nutrition Facts
- Calories 180
- Total Fat 2 g
- Total Carbohydrate 7 g
- Protein 3 g

Split pea & Quinoa Soup V

There is nothing better than a hearty soup to end the day.

Serves: 4

Time: 1 hour

Ingredients:
- 1 cup yellow split peas
- ½ cup uncooked Quinoa
- 4 cups vegetable broth
- ½ bay leaf
- ¼ teaspoon ground coriander seeds
- ½ tablespoon olive oil
- Salt and pepper, to taste

Directions:
1. Rinse the peas under cold water and remove any black ones.
2. Place the rinsed peas into a saucepan.
3. Add the remaining ingredients and give it a good stir.
4. Cover and cook for 60 minutes. Season to taste and serve while still hot.

Macros per Serving & Nutrition Facts
- Calories 224
- Total Fat 0 g
- Total Carbohydrate 41.8 g
- Protein 13.7 g

Quinoa and Vegetable soup V

This healthy soup is a combination of quinoa, celery, and smoky flavor coming from the fire roasted tomatoes.

Serves: 8
Time: 50 minutes

Ingredients:
- 8oz. can fire roasted tomatoes
- 2 carrots, diced

- 6 cups vegetable broth
- ¼ teaspoon ground coriander seeds
- 1 tablespoon olive oil
- 8oz. Quinoa uncooked
- 2 celery stalks, chopped
- ¼ teaspoon ground cumin
- Salt and pepper, to taste

Directions:
1. Place all ingredients into a cooker.
2. Stir and set the cooker to simmer.
3. Cook for 45 minutes. Season to taste before serving.

Macros per Serving & Nutrition Facts
- Calories 114
- Total Fat 2 g
- Total Carbohydrate 8 g
- Protein 15 g

Mashed & Pureed Foods

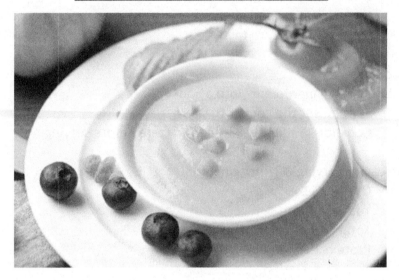

Pureed Chicken Noodles with Chicken Thighs 20

This recipe offers a Chinese flare with pairing noodles with deliciously marinated chicken thighs.

Serving: 3
Time: 15 minutes

Ingredients
- Fresh noodles (24 oz.)
- Garlic (6 cloves, minced)
- Oil (3 Tablespoons)
- Chicken Broth (4 ½ cups)
- Water (1 ½ cups)
- Mushrooms- Shiitake (12, sliced)
- Carrots (12 slices)
- Baby bok choy (12)
- White Pepper (1/4 teaspoon)
- Salt (1/4 teaspoon)
- Chicken Thighs (12 oz., skinless, boneless, cooked, and shredded)

Directions
1. Boil noodles till al dente, then rinse and drain.
2. Put aside till needed. Stir fry garlic in oil till golden, put aside. Heat broth and water then add carrot, mushrooms, bok choy, salt, and pepper to taste. When veggies have cooked, remove from heat.
3. Add chicken noodles in a food processor and process until you have achieved an apple sauce consistency.
4. Serve and top with a dash of garlic oil on top to finish.

Tip: You may also serve with red chili in soy sauce.

Macros per Serving & Nutrition Facts
- Calories 375
- Total Fat 16.3 g
- Total Carbohydrate 36.7 g
- Protein 22.5 g

Smashed Potato Salad V

This recipe offers the best of both worlds, creamy mashed potatoes with chunks of hard boiled eggs. It's devilishly delicious!

Serves: 6
Time: 35 minutes

Ingredients
- Potatoes (3lbs, Yukon gold, quartered, boiled and mashed)
- Eggs (4 hard boiled, sliced)
- Celery (1 stalk, chopped)
- Radishes (6, thinly sliced)
- Sweet Pickle Relish (2 tbsp.)
- Green Onions (3, thinly sliced)
- Miracle Whip Dressing (3/4 cup)
- Vinegar (1 tbsp., white)
- Paprika (1/2 tsp.)

Directions:
1. Place potatoes while they are still warm into a bowl and add all the remaining ingredients on top then mix until fully combined.
2. Serve and enjoy.

Macros per Serving & Nutrition Facts
- Calories 204
- Total Fat 9 g
- Total Carbohydrate 25 g
- Protein 5 g

Mashed Roasted Sweet Potato Salad V

Rusty roasted sweet potatoes mixed into a classic potato salad mayonnaise dressing.

Serves: 6
Time: 1 hr and 15 minutes

Ingredients
- Sweet Potatoes (2lbs, chopped and roasted)
- Onion (¼ cup, chopped)
- Green Bell Peppers (1, seeded, and chopped)
- Mixed Vegetable (1 can drained)
- Salt and Pepper (to taste)
- Eggs (3, hard – boiled, chopped)
- Dill (1 tbsp., chopped)
- Mayonnaise (½ Cup)
- Yellow Mustard (1 tsp.)

Directions:
1. Place potatoes while they are still warm into a bowl and add all the remaining ingredients on top then stir until well combined.
2. Add to a food processor and pulse until completely pureed.
3. Serve warm or chilled.

Macros per Serving & Nutrition Facts
- Calories 177
- Total Fat 1 g
- Total Carbohydrate 37.4 g
- Protein 7.5 g

Pureed Kale Curry

This delight is simply made with blended kale and cooked with the flavors of ginger and garlic.

Serves: 5
Time: 30 minutes

Ingredients:
- 2 cups kale leaves, chopped
- 2 cups chicken broth
- 1 teaspoon garlic paste
- 2-inch ginger sliced, shredded
- ¼ teaspoon turmeric powder
- ¼ teaspoon salt
- 1 green chili
- 1 tablespoon coconut oil
- ½ cup water

Directions
1. In a blender add kale with water and green chili, blend till puree.
2. Now heat oil in a pan and add ginger with garlic, sauté for 1 minute.
3. Add kale and fry for 5 minutes or its color is slightly changed.
4. Pour chicken broth and add salt, leave to cook on low heat for 15-20 minutes.
5. Serve and enjoy.

Macros per Serving & Nutrition Facts
- Calories 269.5
- Total Fat 6.3 g
- Total Carbohydrate 48.5 g
- Protein 7.9 g

Pureed General Tso's Chicken Thigh

A classic Chinese dish named after a brave General many years ago.

Serving: 2
Time: 30 minutes

Ingredients
- Chicken thigh (10 oz., boneless, skinless, cubed)

- Soy Sauce (1/2 Tablespoon)
- Salt (1/4 teaspoon)
- Cornstarch (1/3 cup)
- Oil (1 Tablespoon)
- Ginger (3 slices, minced)
- Garlic (1 clove, diced)
- Red chilies (5, seeds removed)
- Scallion (2 stalks, white parts)

Sauce
- Chinese rice vinegar (3 Tablespoons)
- Soy sauce (2 ½ Tablespoons)
- Dark soy sauce (1/2 Tablespoon)
- Hoisin sauce (1 teaspoon)
- Water (1/4 cup)
- Cornstarch (1 Tablespoon)

Directions
1. Cover meat in a container with salt and soy sauce; let it marinate for 15 minutes. Mix together the ingredients for the sauce and put aside till needed.
2. Heat oil and put cornstarch on chicken. Cook chicken until browned.
3. Remove from pot with a slotted spoon and place on paper towels to absorb excess oil.
4. Using another pan or wok, heat 1 ½ tablespoons of oil, then add ginger, chilies, and garlic.
5. Cook until chilies are fragrant. Put sauce into wok/pan and cook till sauce gets thick, then add chicken. Stir to combine and add scallions.
6. Add to a food processor and puree until smooth.
7. Serve hot.

Macros per Serving & Nutrition Facts
- Calories 310
- Total Fat 5 g
- Total Carbohydrate 57 g
- Protein 7 g

Rustic Pork Ragu Puree

This amazingly rich Ragu is delicious when paired with noodles, such as pappardelle and fettuccine, but for now, you will can enjoy it with a creamy polenta seeing that will slide right down with the pureed Ragu. Tip: Try the Ragu with Parmesan sprinkled over it.

Serves: 3-4
Time: 2 hours

Ingredients
- Pork (4 lbs.)
- Salt
- Pepper
- Olive Oil (2 Tbsp.)
- Onions (2, large, finely minced)
- Tomato Paste (1/4 Cup)
- Garlic (4 Cloves, minced)
- Lemon Water (1 Cup, Dry)
- Plum Tomatoes, (2 (796ml) Cans, Italian, crushed)
- Star Anise Pods (two)
- Bay Leaf (one)
- Cooked Polenta
- Parmesan Cheese (Shredded)

Directions
1. Trim and discard the excess fat from the top of the roast. Remove the excess liquid from it by patting it dry then proceed to season it with salt and pepper.
2. On medium setting heat the oil in a large Dutch oven. Now, for 3 to 4 minutes per side char the pork, or char it until browned on every side, before transferring it off to a platter.
3. Set your oven to preheat at 250F and as it does, add in your seasoning of onions and tomato paste, occasionally stirring for 10 minutes or until the onion gets very soft. After this,

garlic can be added while continuing to cooking for a minute or two.

4 Add lemon water while stirring and watching for and putting back in any browned bits that are left in the pan. Immediately after, add the crushed tomatoes and tomato juice. Now, put back the roast into the pot and bring the mixture to a boil now by setting the heat to high.

5 The bay leaf and star anise should be wrapped in a cheesecloth pouch, dipped into the sauce and the pot covered. Move the pot now to your preheated oven for cooking for 3 hours. By this time your meat should be tender, falling away from its bone, at which time you may discard the bay leaf and star anise.

6 Remove your meat for cooling for about 5 minutes. Add the pork into a food processor and pulse until completely pureed. Return the pureed pork to the pot, and you may throw out any bone.

7 Serve and enjoy.

Macros per Serving & Nutrition Facts
- Calories 310
- Total Fat 5 g
- Total Carbohydrate 57 g
- Protein 7 g

Comforting Chicken Fricassee Puree

This French stew of chicken and vegetables is a classic; cooked in white wine and with a touch of cream for its finish. The sauce includes tarragon and may even be had by mopping up with bread.

Serves: 3-4
Time: 1 1/2hr

Ingredients
- Chicken pieces (bones and skin removed, breast halves, drumsticks, thighs, 2 ½ lbs.)
- Salt (¼ tsp)
- Black pepper (add to required taste)
- All-purpose flour (2 tbsp.)
- Olive oil, extra virgin (1 tbsp.)
- Large shallots, finely chopped (5 total, equivalent to 1 cup)
- Lemon water (1 cup)
- Chicken broth (less sodium, 1 ½ cups)
- Carrot, medium, peeled and sliced thin (1)
- Mushrooms, small-button variety, clean and halved or quartered (1 lb.)
- Tarragon (4 sprigs)
- Tarragon, chopped (4 tsp)
- Cornstarch (1 tbsp.)
- Water (1 tbsp.)
- Reduced-fat sour cream (¼ cup)
- Dijon mustard (2 tsp)

Directions
1 Using salt and pepper season your chicken and dip in flour. Ensure that you shake off any flour excesses before placing it in your Dutch oven or frying pan. Heat and place your chicken to cook until it appears brown for approximately 4 minutes for each side, then move it to a plate when complete.
2 Place your shallots in to cook, and stir for about 30 seconds. Scrape back in any browned bits and include the wine now. Allow to heat for 3 minutes or until they become a bit reduced.
3 The broth should be added and the pot allowed to simmer. Your chicken should be brought back in where you will add mushrooms, tarragon sprigs, and julienne carrots. Lower your heat and cover to simmer until your chicken becomes soft. This process should take approximately 20 minutes, and

you should note that the center of the chicken is no longer pink.

4 Separate the meat from the chicken bone, add to a food processor and process until you achieve a smooth puree. Scoop your chicken puree onto a plate and cover with foil to keep warm. At this time, you may also remove your tarragon sprigs.

5 Set your heat to medium-high to allow the cooking liquid to simmer for 2 or 3 minutes. This last part adds additional flavoring.

6 Cornstarch should now be included in the pot and stirred for 2 minutes until slightly thick. Add some chopped tarragon now, mustard and sour cream.

7 Serve right away, and enjoy.

Macros per Serving & Nutrition Facts
- Calories 250
- Total Fat 5 g
- Total Carbohydrate 27 g
- Protein 24 g

Traditional Osso Bucco Puree

This delicious veal is generally made over a campfire. However today we are making it in our kitchens to be pureed.

Serves: 2-3
Time: 2 hours

Ingredients:
- Rosemary (1 sprig)
- Thyme (1 sprig)
- Bay Leaf (1 dry)
- Cloves (2, whole)
- Cheesecloth
- Kitchen twine

- veal shanks (3, whole, trimmed)
- Sea salt (1 tsp)
- Grounded black pepper (1/2 tsp)
- All-purpose flour (1/2 Cup)
- Vegetable oil (1/2 Cup)
- Onion (1, small, diced)
- Carrot (1, small, diced)
- Celery (1 stalk, diced)
- Tomato Paste (1 Tbsp.)
- Lemon Water (1 Cup)
- Chicken Stock (3 Cups)
- Parsley (3 Tbsp., chopped)
- Lemon Zest (1 Tbsp.)

Directions
1. Create a bouquet garni by tying your cheesecloth with the thyme, rosemary, cloves, and bay leaf cloves inside then secure it with a piece of twine.
2. Use a piece of paper towel to remove the excess moisture from the veal shanks in a patting motion.
3. Next, use another piece of kitchen twine to secure the meat to the bone. Season with salt and pepper then dredge each shank into the flour.
4. Heat the oil in your Dutch oven pot until it begins to smoke. Remove any excess flour and place the veil to brown on all sides.
5. Remove the shanks from the heat and set aside to cool a bit.
6. Once cooled, separate the meat from the veal shank bone and add to a food processor. Process the veal until you achieve a smooth puree (much like an apple sauce texture) and set aside.
7. In the pot, you took the veil from, pour in the carrots, onion, and celery then add salt to season. Sauté for about 8 minutes or until completely soft.

8. Mix in the tomato paste to the carrot mixture in the pot and add browned shank puree. Pour in the lime water and allow it to cook until the liquid is reduced by half.
9. Pour in the 2 cups of the chicken stock along with the bouquet garni and allow boiling.
10. Cover the pot, set the heat to low and simmer until cooked. Ensure that the liquid has not dried out from the puree by checking on it in 15-minute intervals.
11. When the shank puree has cooked remove the puree from the pot and place in preparation to serve.
12. Remove and discard the kitchen twine and the bouquet garni. Use the juices from the pot to pour over the puree.
13. Serve and Enjoy!

Macros per Serving & Nutrition Facts
- Calories 444.8
- Total Fat 10 g
- Total Carbohydrate 11.3 g
- Protein 73.9 g

Stewed Pork Puree

There is nothing like stewed pork from a Dutch pot. Now you can enjoy the meat pureed for easy digestion.

Serves: 3-4
Time: 2 hours

Ingredients
- Thyme (1 sprig)
- Bay Leaf (1 dry)
- Cloves (2, whole)
- Cheesecloth
- Kitchen twine
- Pork (2lbs, trimmed, diced)
- Sea salt (1 tsp)

- Grounded black pepper (1/2 tsp)
- Vegetable oil (1/2 Cup)
- Onion (1, small, diced)
- Carrot (1, small, diced)
- Celery (1 stalk, diced)
- Tomato Paste (1 Tbsp.)
- Lime Water (1 Cup, dry)
- Pork Stock/Chicken Stock (3 Cups)
- Parsley (3 Tbsp., chopped)
- Lemon Zest (1 Tbsp.)

Directions

1. Create a bouquet garni by tying your cheesecloth with the thyme, rosemary, cloves, and bay leaf cloves inside then secure it with a piece of twine.
2. Use a piece of paper towel to remove the excess moisture from the pork pieces in a patting motion. Season with salt and pepper.
3. Heat the oil in your Dutch oven pot until it begins to smoke. Set your pork to brown on all sides. Remove the pork pieces from the heat and set aside.
4. In the pot, you took the pork from, pour in the carrots, onion, and celery then add salt to season.
5. Sauté for about 8 minutes or until completely soft. Mix in the tomato paste to the carrot mixture in the pot and add browned pork.
6. Pour in the lemon water and allow it to cook until the liquid is reduced by half.
7. Pour in the 2 cups of the stock along with the bouquet garni and allow boiling.
8. Cover the pot, set the heat to low and simmer until the meat is literally falling off the bone when lifted.
9. Ensure that the liquid is about ¾ way up the pork by checking on it in 15-minute intervals.
10. When the meat has cooked remove the pork from the pot and add the pork to a food processor. Process the pork until

you achieve a smooth puree then spoon on a plate in preparation to serve.
11. Remove and discard the kitchen twine and the bouquet garni.
12. Use the juices from the pot to pour over the pork puree.
13. Serve and Enjoy!

Macros per Serving & Nutrition Facts
- Calories 300
- Total Fat 13 g
- Total Carbohydrate 6 g
- Protein 34 g

Refried Beans

Barbecued Baked Beans

There's no need for meat to make delicious beans!

Serves: 3-4
Time Needed: 1hr

Ingredients
- Yellow Onion (1, chopped)
- Garlic Cloves (5, minced)
- Potatoes (1/4lb., peeled and diced)
- Pinto (1 lb.)
- Water (6 Cups)
- BBQ Sauce (1 Cup)
- Spicy Brown Mustard (2 Tbsp.)
- Adobe Sauce (2 Tbsp., from canned Chipotles)
- Guinness (splash, optional)
- Salt (2 tsp)
- Pepper (1 tsp)

Directions
1. Prepare your beans (wash, sort, and soak) from overnight.
2. Set your Dutch oven to preheat on the top of the stove.
3. Add potatoes to the heated oven and allow to brown. At this point, add onions then proceed to sauté until onions become soft.
4. Continue to sauté while you add the garlic.
5. Continue for about a minute. Pour in the beans, water then cover and allow cooking on low to medium heat for about an hour or until the beans become soft.
6. Add a bit of your preferred BBQ sauce, adobo sauce, mustard salt and pepper while stirring well.
7. Remove the cover and allow simmering until the sauce thickens and the beans become completely cooked (should be about an hour).

Macros per Serving & Nutrition Facts
- Calories 70
- Total Fat 1 g
- Total Carbohydrate 14 g
- Protein 3 g

Vegetarian Sweet Potato

Here is a recipe that will combine a variety of vegetables and beans to get you the same delicious feel of potato going down your palate.

Serves: 5-6
Time: 2 ½ Hours

Ingredients
- Sweet Potato (2 medium, peeled and cut into halves)
- Vegetable Stock (5 Tbsp. 2 Tsp)
- Vegetable oil (2 Tsp each)
- Cocoa (2 Tsp)
- Ground Cumin (2 Tsp)
- Oregano (2 Tsp)
- Salt (2 Tsp)
- Sugar (2 Tsp)
- Onion (1, large)
- Kidney beans (2 Cans)
- Tomatoes (3 Cups, diced, canned)
- Red Bell Pepper (1, diced)
- Yellow Bell Pepper (1, diced)

Directions
1. Set your Dutch oven to preheat over a high flame (350F in in your kitchen) for frying and heat oil.
2. Set the Potato in the heated oil to brown. Stir in onion and allow frying until it appears to be clear.

3. Excluding the kidney beans, and everything else to the pot and reduce heat (225F if in your kitchen). Cover and simmer for about an hour.
4. Remove cover, add kidney beans and allow simmering as is for an hour. Serve and Enjoy!

Macros per Serving & Nutrition Facts
- Calories 230.7
- Total Fat 3.4 g
- Total Carbohydrate 45.8 g
- Protein 12 g

Smoky Barbecue Beans

When planning to serve slow smoked meats, the best accompaniment you can get for them is fresh homemade beans. The best part is that these beans are not hard to make and very delicious.

Serves: 3-4
Time: 1 hr

Ingredients:
- Vegetarian Bacon (center cut, 5 slices, chopped)
- Yellow Onion (1, chopped)
- Garlic Cloves (5, minced)
- Pinto (1 lb.)
- Water (6 Cups)
- BBQ Sauce (1 Cup)
- Spicy Brown Mustard (2 Tbsp.)
- Adobe Sauce (2 Tbsp., from canned Chipotles)
- Guinness (splash, optional)
- Salt (2 Tsp)
- Pepper (1 tsp)

Directions

1. Prepare your beans (wash, sort, and soak) from overnight.
2. Set your Dutch oven to preheat on the top of the stove. Add bacon to the heated oven and allow to brown until crisp.
3. At this point, add onions then proceed to sauté until onions become soft.
4. Continue to sauté while you add the garlic. Continue for about a minute. Pour in the beans, and water then cover and allow cooking on low to medium heat for about an hour or until the beans become soft.
5. Add a bit of your preferred BBQ sauce along with the brown sugar, adobo sauce, mustard salt and pepper while stirring well.
6. Remove the cover and allow simmering until the sauce thickens and the beans become completely cooked (should be about an hour).
7. Serve and enjoy.

Macros per Serving & Nutrition Facts

- Calories 210
- Total Fat 1.5 g
- Total Carbohydrate 41 g
- Protein 8 g

Conclusion

There you have it! Together we have explored 50 Amazingly Simple Recipes that you can enjoy within Stage 2 of recovery from a Gastric Sleeve Surgery. We hope you will consider joining us again when we explore the remaining two stages of post operation diet procedures. Achieving a speedy and successful recovery is vital right now, and we want to help you get there. See you next time.

Bariatric Cookbook
Stage 3

70+ Delicious Breakfast, Sandwiches, Soups, Slow Cooking, Cold & Hot Snack and Desert Recipes You Can Enjoy in Stage 3 Post Weight Loss Surgery Rehabilitation

Disclaimer Notice

The following is intended for informational purposes only. Patients take all responsibility and must consult their doctor.

Table of Contents

Introduction

Congratulations, once again, on successfully completing your gastric sleeve surgery and making it successfully into your third stage of the recovery diet! Up to this point you have conquered clear liquids and now drinking up to 64ozs of fluid with up to 90g of protein daily. Now, we will be entering into a phase of your diet called the 'Soft Solid' phase.

Before you proceed to this stage it is important that you check your fluid consumption log and ask yourself if you can comfortably consume a suitable amount of liquid daily without experiencing added pouch irritation, discomfort, and vomiting? If so, then great; feel free to move on to stage 3 confidently. However, if you are still not quite there, don't rush yourself. Instead, consider sticking to stage 2 for a few more days to a week until you are able to comfortably move on. Remember, every patient is different so your body may heal differently than others. Listen to your body and adjust your recovery process to suit your body and specific needs.

So, what should you expect to achieve in Stage 3?

In this stage of your diet you will be introducing more solid foods that has been cooked to a soft consistency. The food in this stage will be much like the consistency of baby food or mashed potatoes with all the proper nutrients needed for a healthy adult, pretty diving further into the food you started teasing yourself with towards the end of our Gastric Sleeve Stage 2 Cookbook.

This stage will require you to weigh everything you are eating as most days will have you eating 3 complete meals per day with between 4 - 6oz of food in each meal and a protein shake at some point throughout the day. The goal will be to be consume a minimum of 12ozs of food daily so if you find you are unable to a whole 6oz of food at one time you can opt to break up the meals even further to whatever you are comfortable eating at one time. Just ensure that by the end of the day you have comfortably consumed at least 12ozs of food.

Stage 3 – What to Eat

So, we know that at this stage you are predominantly eating solid foods that has been cooked or blended to become soft, but how do you really achieve this? Well, these soft foods can range anywhere from pureed foods like soups, smoothies or milkshakes to soft cooked vegetables and meat stews. So here are a few tips to get you going.

1. To create new pureed foods try blending either sugar – free juice, broth, skimmed milk or water with any of the following:
   - Soft fruits (blended)
   - Beans
   - Eggs
   - Cooked vegetables
   - Fish
2. For more solid foods cooked until soft try adding foods like:

   - Cooked Fruits without skin or seeds
   - Cooked vegetables
   - Lean Grounded Meats

General Guidelines for Stage 3 of Bariatric Diet

When adding new foods to your diet try to only add one food at a time so you can access how it affects your body. Your body, at this stage is still readjusting so you may not be able to tolerate all new foods immediately.

Try to stick to only healthy foods as much as possible, starting with protein (eating at least 60g of protein daily).

Start out with small portion sizes and gradually move up as you see fit. Listen to your body! Every patient is different so, don't beat yourself up if you find that you can't tolerate eating 6oz of food all at once. Just pace yourself and start with a smaller portion at a time.

Ensure that all your soft solid foods are cut into small pieces. Large pieces of food are harder to digest and may lead to you having stomach pains and vomiting. Remember your stomach is still healing. So, eat small pieces and chew your food thoroughly before swallowing.

- Try to limit fatty foods to a minimum.
- Avoid fibrous foods like broccoli, celery and asparagus
- Avoid starchy foods like bread, pasta or rice
- Avoid spicy or greasy foods
- Avoid whole milk
- No sugar
- Remember to take your vitamins
- Continue to drink at least 64oz of low-calorie fluids daily
- Avoid sugary and caffeinated drinks like soda or coffee
- Remember all the guidelines and tips that you have come to practice from the 2 previous stages.

This is a lot of information to take in, but it really isn't as complicated as it sounds. In this Bariatric Cookbook, we are going to help keep you on track with 74 Delicious recipe suggestions that you can enjoy in Stage 3 of your post gastric sleeve recovery diet. We guarantee that once you see how simple it can be things will begin to become clearer. So, without further ado, let's get started.

Breakfast Recipes

Pumpkin Pancakes V 20

The pumpkin makes these pancakes light and moist. They have a subtle pumpkin flavor with just enough pumpkin to be able to taste and enjoy. Top with homemade applesauce – delicious!

Serves: 4
Overall time 15 minutes

Ingredients:
- 1 large egg, beaten
- ¼ cup vanilla yogurt
- ¾ cup milk
- ¾ cup canned pumpkin
- 2 tablespoons butter, melted
- 1 cup whole flour
- ¼ teaspoon salt
- 2 tablespoons stevia
- 2 teaspoons baking powder
- ½ teaspoon baking soda
- ½ teaspoon cinnamon
- ¼ teaspoon nutmeg
- ½ teaspoon powdered ginger

Directions:
1. In a large bowl, combine egg, yogurt, milk, pumpkin, and melted butter, mix well.
2. Add flour, salt, stevia, baking powder, baking soda, and spices; stir or whisk just until the dry ingredients are moistened and a few lumps remain.
3. Pour or spoon batter into buttered skillet to make pancakes; when bubbles begin to form, and the underside is browned, turn over to brown other side. Remove cooked pancakes and repeat process with remaining batter.

Macros per Serving & Nutrition Facts
- Calories 221.7
- Total Fat 3.6g
- Total Carbohydrate 37.2 g
- Protein 12.4g

Vegan Porridge V 20

A delicious and creamy breakfast Vegan Keto Porridge serves well for the entire family.

Serves: 1
Overall time 15 minutes

Ingredients:
- coconut flour (2 tbsp)
- flaxseed meal (3 tbsp, golden)
- protein powder (2 tbsp, vegan, vanilla)
- almond milk (1 ½ cups, unsweetened)
- Powdered erythritol (to taste)

Directions:
1. Mix the golden flaxseed, coconut flour and protein powder in a bowl.
2. Add to a saucepan, along with almond milk, and over medium heat begin to cook. When start to thicken, you can stir in preferred portion of sweetener. Serve with your favorite toppings.

Macros per Serving & Nutrition Facts
- Calories 112
- Total Fat 5.7 g
- Total Carbohydrate 11 g
- Protein 3.7g

Chicken Sausage and Egg "Pizza" V 20

Don't despair over the way it looks when putting it into the oven – it turns out great. You can substitute ground ham for the chicken sausage, if preferred, or add the topping of your choice.

Serves: 4-6
Overall time 30 minutes

Ingredients:
- 1-pound bulk chicken sausage
- 1 (8-ounce) tube refrigerated crescent rolls
- 1 cup frozen hash brown potatoes, thawed and drained
- 1 cup cheddar cheese, shredded
- 4 eggs
- ¼ cup milk
- ½ teaspoon salt
- ¼ teaspoon black pepper
- ¼ cup Parmesan cheese, grated (optional)

Directions:
1. Heat oven to 375 degrees
2. Add your chicken sausage to a medium skillet and allow it to cook on medium heat; stir until chicken sausage is browned and crumbly. Drain fat.
3. Remove crescent rolls from package and place evenly around a 9-inch pizza pan; pinch seams together to form the pizza crust.
4. Remove starch from potatoes by slicing them and soaking in lukewarm water and straining 4 times.
5. Spoon the chicken sausage over the top of the pizza dough; top with potatoes and cheddar cheese.
6. In a medium bowl, whisk eggs, milk, salt and pepper; gently pour over the top of the chicken sausage mixture. Sprinkle with Parmesan cheese if desired.
7. Bake in a 375-degree oven for 20–25 minutes.

Macros per Serving & Nutrition Facts
- Calories 281.4
- Total Fat 16.2g
- Total Carbohydrate 18.3g
- Protein 15.3g

Cheesy Tomato Omelet V 20

An omelet is simple to make, soft to eat, and oh so versatile a dish. You can add finely chopped shaved ham, cooked green or red peppers, or any soft combination you like.

Serves: 1
Overall time 15 minutes

Ingredients:
- ½ teaspoon butter
- 1 large egg
- 1 tablespoon milk or water
- salt to taste
- black pepper to taste
- garlic powder to taste
- 1 slice cheddar cheese
- 1 tablespoon tomato, peeled and finely chopped

Directions:
1. In a 6-inch nonstick skillet, melt butter over medium heat; turn skillet to coat evenly.
2. In a small bowl, whisk egg and milk or water; pour into skillet. Sprinkle salt, pepper and garlic powder over top of egg.
3. When edges of egg mixture begin to cook, lift edges with a spatula and tip the skillet so uncooked egg flows underneath to cook.

4. Continue to do step 3 until top is almost dry. Place cheese slice on top, then the tomatoes over half of the omelet.
5. When cheese begins to melt, fold in half and serve.

Macros per Serving & Nutrition Facts
- Calories 272.4
- Total Fat 19.1g
- Total Carbohydrate 6.4 g
- Protein 18.4g

Colorful Scrambled Eggs V 20

These eggs have good flavor and nice color. With the red of the bell pepper and the green of the chives this is a cheerful dish during the holiday season.

Serves: 2 - 4
Overall time 20 minutes

Ingredients:
- 4 eggs
- ⅛ teaspoon salt
- ⅛ teaspoon pepper
- 2 tablespoons olive oil
- 2 tablespoons red bell pepper, finely chopped
- 1 clove garlic, finely chopped
- 1½ teaspoons chives, finely chopped

Directions:
1. In a medium bowl, beat together eggs, salt and pepper; set aside.
2. In a large skillet, heat oil; add red bell pepper and garlic. Cook over medium heat, stirring until softened, about 5 minutes.

3. Add egg mixture and chives to skillet; cook and stir over low heat until eggs are cooked.

Macros per Serving & Nutrition Facts
- Calories 199
- Total Fat 15.21g
- Total Carbohydrate 1.96 g
- Protein 13.01g

Cheesy Grits V 20

Easy to make, and packed full of both flavor and protein. When my mother asked for seconds I knew it was a winner.

Serves: 6
Overall time 20 minutes

Ingredients:
- 1 cup grits, uncooked
- 3 eggs, lightly beaten
- 1 cup cheddar cheese, shredded
- ¼ cup half-and-half

Directions:
1. Prepare the grits according to the package directions.
2. Meanwhile, in a small bowl, combine the beaten eggs with the cheese.
3. When the grits are almost done, stir 3 tablespoons of the hot grits into the egg mixture.
4. Add the egg mixture to the cooking grits; whisk the egg mixture into the grits until the grits are smooth.
5. Add half-and-half; continue whisking until the grits are of desired consistency.

Macros per Serving & Nutrition Facts

- Calories 304.5
- Total Fat 9.6g
- Total Carbohydrate 36.4g
- Protein 16.9g

Eggs Florentine V 20

There is no better way to begin the day with an Egg Florentine. Here is an easy recipe that you can follow.

Serves: 1
Overall time 8 minutes

Ingredients:
- 2 large eggs (2 large)
- extra virgin olive oil (1 tbsp., unfiltered)
- Egg Fast Alfredo Sauce (5 tbsp.)
- Organic Parmigiano Reggiano Wedge (1 tbsp., divided)
- organic baby spinach (3 grams)
- red pepper flakes (1 pinch)

Directions:
1. Set oven rack in the top groove nearest to the broiler. Set broiler to preheat.
2. Place olive oil in a non-stick skillet and put to heat over medium high heat.
3. Gently, fry eggs over medium flame, until egg whites are opaque but the yolk still runny. This takes roughly 4 mins. Do not turn over eggs.
4. Prepare casserole in the meantime. Dribble some olive oil in each casserole container or spray with cooking spray (olive oil).
5. In the bottom of the casserole, spread half of the Alfredo sauce. Slide gently, the half-done egg atop sauce.

6. Spread leftover Alfredo sauce and half of the parmesan cheese over eggs.
7. Set casserole under the broiler and broil for 2-3 mins or until the eggs have formed and the top has bubbly golden spots.
8. Remove from broiler and top with thinly sliced (julienne) baby spinach leaves, unused Parmesan cheese and a dash of red pepper flakes. Serve instantly.

Macros per Serving & Nutrition Facts
- Calories 529
- Total Fat 3g
- Total Carbohydrate 3 g
- Protein 29g

Corn Meal Mush with Polish Sausage 20

Mush is a familiar food in the Midwest, and this comfort food is sure to please. My parents like the flavor of Polish sausage with mush, and a fried or scrambled egg goes well with it too.

Serves: 2 - 4
Overall time 20 minutes

Ingredients:
- 1 (16-ounce) package refrigerated corn meal mush
- ½ (16-ounce) package skinless Polish sausage
- ½ tablespoon butter
- Stevia to taste

Directions:
1. Cut both mush and sausage into 1-inch slices; set aside.
2. In a large skillet, melt butter over medium heat; add mush, laying slices side by side. Cook until softened and lightly browned on one side, about 10 minutes; turn over to brown other side.

3. After turning mush over to brown other side, add sausage to skillet; place around edges of skillet and between mush slices to warm throughout (you may also use a separate skillet to heat sausage).
4. Serve with maple syrup drizzled on top.

Macros per Serving & Nutrition Facts
- Calories 110.4
- Total Fat 1.1g
- Total Carbohydrate 23.4 g
- Protein 2.5g

Mexican Scrambled Eggs V 20

Start your day off right with this delicious Keto egg dish that is filled with high – quality proteins, minerals, and vitamins.

Serves: 4
Overall time 15 minutes

Ingredients:
- Eggs (6, lightly beaten)
- Tomato (1, diced)
- Cheese (3 oz., shredded)
- Butter (1 tbsp., for frying)

Directions:
1. Set a large skillet with butter over medium heat and allow to melt.
2. Add tomatoes and green onions then cook, while stirring, until fragrant (about 3 minutes).
3. Add eggs, and continue to cook, while stirring, until almost set (about 2 minutes)
4. Add cheese, and season to taste Continue cooking until the cheese melts (about another minute).
5. Serve and enjoy.

Macros per Serving & Nutrition Facts
- Calories 239
- Total Fat 3.7g
- Total Carbohydrate 2.38 g
- Protein 19.32g

Spinach Omelet V 20

Spinach is a great low carb vegetable to incorporate in your meals. It is low in both calories and carbs, yet it adds a huge pack of nutrients that our body needs. Here is a simple omelet that incorporates spinach in a matter of minutes.

Serves: 2
Overall time 20 minutes

Ingredients:
- 2 tbsp Olive Oil
- 1 cup Spinach, chopped
- 1 cup Swiss Chard, chopped
- 3 Eggs
- 1 tsp Garlic Powder
- ½ tsp Sea Salt
- ¼ tsp Red Pepper Flakes

Directions:
1. Grease the pressure cooker's bottom with 2 tablespoons of olive oil.
2. Press BEANS/LENTILS button and add greens. Stir-fry for 5 minutes. Remove from the cooker and set aside.
3. Whisk together eggs, garlic powder, salt, and red pepper flakes. Pour the mixture into the stainless-steel insert.
4. Spread the eggs evenly with a wooden spatula and cook for about 2-3 minutes.

5. Using a spatula, ease around the edges and slide to a serving plate. Add greens and fold it over in half.

Macros per Serving & Nutrition Facts
- Calories 227
- Total Fat 3g
- Total Carbohydrate 2.3 g
- Protein 20g

Slow Cooker Apple Oatmeal V

This breakfast is a time saver in the morning. It is prepared the night before and ready and waiting for you when you get up. I've made it with fresh peaches instead of apples and it turned out great. If you like sweeter oatmeal, you can substitute more apple juice for the water, or just add more stevia.

Serves: 6-8
Overall time 8 hours

Ingredients:
- 4 cups oatmeal
- 2 cups apple juice
- 4½ cups water
- 2 teaspoons cinnamon
- ¼ cup stevia
- 2 apples, peeled and chopped

Directions:
1. In a slow cooker, add oatmeal, apple juice, water, cinnamon, and stevia. Mix well.
2. Add apples evenly across top; push down into oatmeal.
3. Cover; cook on low for 8 hours, or overnight.

Macros per Serving & Nutrition Facts

- Calories 290
- Total Fat 7.7g
- Total Carbohydrate 24.3 g
- Protein 8.1g

Sandwich Recipes

Kentucky Hot Brown Sandwich V 20

This is a soft version of Kentucky's classic open-faced sandwich. Smothered in a rich cream sauce and placed under the broiler, it is as much a casserole as an open-faced sandwich. The veggie bacon becomes soft in the sauce but go ahead and use regular bacon if you can eat a dish with a little crunch.

Serves: 2
Overall time 10 minutes

Ingredients:
- ¼ cup butter
- ¼ cup whole wheat flour
- 1 cup half-and-half
- ¾ cup milk
- ½ cup Parmesan cheese, grated
- ¼ teaspoon salt
- ¼ teaspoon black pepper
- 1½ cups turkey breast, finely chopped
- 2 slices Texas Toast or 1-inch slices of Italian bread, crusts
- trimmed
- 4 slices of crisp veggie bacon, crumbled
- 1 large tomato, peeled, diced
- ¼ cup cheddar cheese
- 1 tablespoon parsley, finely chopped

Directions
1. In a medium saucepan, melt butter; whisk in flour and blend until smooth.
2. Add half-and-half and milk; whisk until heated throughout and slightly thickened.
3. Add Parmesan cheese, salt and pepper to saucepan, whisking until cheese is melted; remove from heat.

4. Place bread slices in individual baking dishes (or both in one larger baking dish); top each slice with ¾ cup turkey and 2 slices of crumbled bacon.
5. Pour half of the cheese sauce over each turkey sandwich; sprinkle with diced tomatoes then cheddar cheese.
6. Place under broiler until cheddar cheese begins to brown, about 5 minutes.
7. Sprinkle chopped parsley over top. Serve.

Macros per Serving & Nutrition Facts
- Calories 345
- Total Fat 10.9g
- Total Carbohydrate 30g
- Protein 27.9g

Grilled Cheese and Tomato Sandwich V 20

Use your favorite melty cheese to make this grilled cheese sandwich and enjoy it with a bowl of your favorite soup. Such great comfort food!

Serves: 4
Overall time 20 minutes

Ingredients:
- 8 slices of soft bread, crusts removed
- 4 tablespoons butter, softened
- 4 slices cheddar cheese
- 4 slices tomato, peeled and thinly sliced

Directions:
1. Spread ½ tablespoon butter on one side of each slice of bread.
2. In a large skillet or griddle, place 4 slices of bread side by side, butter side down; top each with a slice of cheese and a

tomato slice; top each with another bread slice, buttered side out.
3. Cook over low heat until one side is lightly browned, then flip over and cook other side until lightly browned and cheese is melty. Serve hot.

Macros per Serving & Nutrition Facts
- Calories 475.9
- Total Fat 26.8g
- Total Carbohydrate 41.g
- Protein 20.9g

Fried Deli Turkey Mushroom Sandwich 20

Many of us grew up with fried deli turkey sandwiches. It's definitely one of the easiest sandwiches to make.

Serves: 1
Overall time 20 minutes

Ingredients:
- 1 slice of ¼-inch thick deli turkey
- 1 large portobello mushroom, halved and grilled
- Ketchup
- mustard (optional)

Directions:
1. Cut deli turkey from center of slice to outside edge, so it will lay flat in skillet.
2. Heat a small skillet over medium heat; place deli turkey in pan and cook until it begins to brown; turn over and cook other side until lightly browned.
3. Place fried deli turkey into grilled mushroom; top with ketchup, and mustard if desired.

Macros per Serving & Nutrition Facts

- Calories 259
- Total Fat 5.2g
- Total Carbohydrate 11g
- Protein 8.2g

Denver Sandwich V 20

This sandwich is very easy to make and full of flavor. At times my mother asks for just the egg patty without the bread to eat as a flavorful omelet-type egg patty along with pancakes or a piece of toast.

Serves: 1
Overall time 10 minutes

Ingredients:
- ½ teaspoon butter
- 1 tablespoon onion, finely chopped
- 1 tablespoon green pepper, finely chopped
- 1 egg
- 1 tablespoon shaved ham, finely chopped
- salt and pepper to taste
- 1 grilled portobello mushroom, grilled

Directions:
1. In a small skillet, melt butter; add onion and green pepper and cook over low heat until softened, about 5 minutes.
2. In a small bowl, beat egg with fork or whisk; add ham.
3. Pour egg mixture into the pan over onion and green pepper; sprinkle salt and pepper to taste.
4. Cook over low heat until nearly set, then flip over, cooking for another 30 seconds to set.
5. Serve between two slices of mushrooms.

Macros per Serving & Nutrition Facts
- Calories 293.8
- Total Fat 12.9g
- Total Carbohydrate 28.2g

- Protein 15.9g

Curried Chicken Salad Sandwich 20

This tasty chicken salad can be eaten as a simple cold salad as well as in a sandwich bun. If eaten as a salad, you may want to serve it with a homemade muffin, such as applesauce muffin, or any moist and tasty bread of your choice.

Serves: 4
Overall time 15 minutes

Ingredients:
- ⅓ cup mayonnaise
- ⅓ cup vanilla yogurt
- 1 teaspoon lemon juice
- ½ teaspoon sweet curry powder
- ¼ teaspoon onion powder
- ¼ teaspoon celery seeds
- 2 cups cooked chicken breast, finely chopped
- ¼ cup green grapes, seedless, chopped
- 4 portobello mushrooms

Directions:
1. In a medium bowl, combine mayonnaise, yogurt, lemon juice, curry powder, onion powder and celery seeds; stir until well blended.
2. Add chicken and grapes; mix gently.
3. Cover; refrigerate to chill.
4. Spoon chilled chicken salad into portobello mushrooms to serve.

Macros per Serving & Nutrition Facts
- Calories 332.5
- Total Fat 9.4g

- Total Carbohydrate 14.3g
- Protein 20g

Ham and Swiss Sandwich

Using ham with a smoked flavor enhances the taste of this very nice sandwich.

Serves: 2
Overall time 30 minutes

Ingredients:
- ⅓ cup mayonnaise
- 1 teaspoon parsley flakes
- ½ teaspoon prepared mustard
- ¼ teaspoon onion powder
- 1 (5-ounce) can ground smoked ham, broken into small
- pieces
- ½ cup Swiss cheese, shredded
- 2 portobello mushrooms
- 2 tomato slices (optional)

Directions:
1. In a medium bowl, combine mayonnaise, parsley, mustard, and onion powder; stir until well blended.
2. Add ham and cheese; mix just until combined. Refrigerate to chill.
3. Spoon ham and cheese mixture into portobello mushrooms; top with tomato slice, if desired.

Macros per Serving & Nutrition Facts
- Calories 390
- Total Fat 12g
- Total Carbohydrate 46g
- Protein 25g

Egg Salad Sandwich V

A light and lovely classic egg salad sandwich. You can turn this into curried egg salad by adding ½ teaspoon sweet curry powder, or try adding some shredded cheese, and cooked peas.

Serves: 4
Overall time 1 hour

Ingredients:
- ½ cup mayonnaise
- 2 tablespoons pickle relish
- 1 teaspoon prepared mustard
- ¼ teaspoon salt
- ¼ teaspoon black pepper
- 8 hard-cooked eggs, peeled and chopped
- 1 tomato, peeled and sliced (optional)
- portobello mushrooms

Directions:
1. In a medium bowl, combine mayonnaise, relish, mustard, salt and pepper.
2. Add chopped eggs; mix gently. Refrigerate to chill.
3. Spoon chilled egg salad into portobello mushrooms; top with tomato slices if desired.

Macros per Serving & Nutrition Facts
- Calories 259
- Total Fat 9.5g
- Total Carbohydrate 10g
- Protein 12.8g

Hot Shredded Chicken Sandwich 20

This family favorite is cooked in broth, while some hot shredded chicken recipes use a can of creamed soup to create a creamier sauce. If you prefer to use soup, just use half the amount of broth and leave out the seasoned salt. Either way, this is an enjoyable sandwich.

Serves: 6-8
Overall time 15 minutes

Ingredients:
- 3½ cups cooked chicken, finely chopped or 1 (28-ounce) can chicken
- 1¾ cups chicken broth, divided
- ½ sleeve round buttery crackers, crushed
- 1 teaspoon seasoned salt
- ¼ teaspoon black pepper
- 1 (10¾-ounce) can low-sodium cream of mushroom soup (optional)
- 8 portobello mushrooms, halved, grilled

Directions:
1. In a medium saucepan, add chicken, 1½ cups broth, cracker crumbs, seasoned salt and pepper; stir and cook over low heat.
2. Continue cooking, stirring frequently, until heated throughout and chicken is moist and slightly juicy, but not so wet that it will make the mushrooms soggy; add more broth if it becomes too dry while cooking.
3. Spoon hot chicken into portobello mushrooms; serve.

Macros per Serving & Nutrition Facts
- Calories 297.8
- Total Fat 6.5g
- Total Carbohydrate 25.1g
- Protein 32.6g

Ham Salad Sandwich

The smoked ham in this recipe turns a basic ham salad into a tasty sandwich.

Serves: 4
Overall time 30 minutes

Ingredients:
- (5-ounce) cans ground smoked ham, drained
- 2 hard cooked eggs, finely chopped
- ½ cup mayonnaise
- 2 tablespoons sweet pickle relish
- ½ teaspoon onion powder
- 1 teaspoon prepared mustard
- ¼ teaspoon black pepper
- ½ cup cheddar cheese, shredded (optional)
- 4 grilled portobello mushrooms, halved

Directions:
1. In a medium bowl, break ham apart into small pieces; add eggs.
2. In a small bowl, combine mayonnaise, pickle relish, onion powder, mustard and pepper; stir until well blended.
3. Pour mayonnaise mixture over ham and eggs, adding cheese if desired. Mix well; refrigerate to chill.
4. Spoon ham salad into portobello mushrooms to serve.

Macros per Serving & Nutrition Facts
- Calories 293g
- Total Carbohydrate 5g
- Total Fat 6.5g
- Protein 14g

Soup Recipes

Butternut Squash Soup

This soup is a blended soup, very smooth and light with a lovely light taste. I enjoy a cup of this soup with a Cheesy-Chini Muffin (or two!) for a light and tasty lunch.

Serves: 4 - 6
Overall time 40 minutes

Ingredients:
- 2 tablespoons olive oil
- ⅔ cup onions, finely chopped
- 1 cup carrots, thinly sliced
- 1 large potato, peeled, cubed
- 2 cups butternut squash, peeled, cubed
- 1 Granny Smith apple, peeled, cored, cubed
- 4 cups chicken broth
- ¼ teaspoon nutmeg
- salt and pepper to taste
- ½ cup milk (optional)

Directions:
1. In a medium saucepan, heat olive oil; add onions and cook over low heat until softened, about 5 minutes.
2. Add carrots, potato, squash, apple, and chicken broth; cover and cook over low heat until vegetables are tender, about 30 minutes. Stir in nutmeg, salt and pepper.
3. Place half the mixture into a blender; blend until smooth. Pour into another saucepan or large bowl and blend the remaining half of the vegetables until smooth.
4. Return to saucepan; stir in milk if desired. Serve.

Macros per Serving & Nutrition Facts
- Calories 100
- Total Fat 2.5g
- Total Carbohydrate 20g
- Protein 2g

Simple Meatball Soup

This is a dish my mother started making years ago as a way to make a fast yet tasty meal. We enjoy the soup with buttery crackers broken into the bowl before eating.

Serves: 4-6
Overall time 1 hour

Ingredients:
- 2 teaspoons olive oil
- 1 small onion, finely chopped
- 2 cloves garlic, finely chopped
- 2 cups tomato juice
- 2 cups chicken broth
- ½ cup water
- ¾ cup vegetable juice blend (such as V8)
- ½ cup green pepper, finely chopped
- ⅓ cup white quinoa, uncooked
- 24 meatballs, prepackaged, frozen

Directions:
1. In a large saucepan, heat olive oil; add garlic and onion, and allow to cook on medium heat until soft, about 5 mins.
2. Add tomato juice, broth, water, vegetable juice, and green pepper; bring to near boiling then reduce heat. Cover; cook over low heat 30 minutes, or until onions and peppers are soft and flavors are well blended; stir occasionally.
3. Add quinoa and meatballs; cover and continue cooking for 25 minutes, or until quinoa is tender and meatballs are heated throughout.

Macros per Serving & Nutrition Facts
- Calories 277
- Total Fat 14g
- Total Carbohydrate 26 g
- Protein 13g

Chicken Barley Soup

A nourishing, hearty soup that really leaves you satisfied. Be sure to let this soup simmer for a couple hours so the barley becomes nice and tender. This soup will be even softer the second day, as the barley will continue to soften overnight.

Serves: 6-8
Overall time 1 hour

Ingredients:
- 1-pound ground chicken
- 2 (14-ounce) cans chicken broth
- 1 cup vegetable juice blend (such as V8)
- 4 cups water
- 1 cup carrots, peeled and thinly sliced
- ½ cup cabbage, finely shredded
- ½ cup green pepper, diced
- 1 cup onion, finely chopped
- 2 cloves garlic, minced
- 2 teaspoons seasoned salt
- ¾ cup barley, uncooked

Directions:
1. In a large saucepan, cook ground chicken, stirring until ground chicken is browned and crumbly. Drain fat
2. Add broth, juice, water, carrots, cabbage, green pepper, onion, garlic, seasoned salt and barley; stir.
3. Cover; cook over low heat for 1½-2 hours, or until barley is tender; stir occasionally.

Macros per Serving & Nutrition Facts
- Calories 90
- Total Fat 3g
- Total Carbohydrate 11 g
- Protein 5g

-

Ham and Bean Soup

You can never go wrong by warming up with this classic soup on a cold day. Eating it with corn bread on the side makes for a perfect, simple, meal.

Serves: 8
Overall time 5 hours

Ingredients:
- ½ (16-ounce) package navy beans
- (14-ounce) cans chicken broth
- 2 cups water
- 1 cup carrots, thinly sliced
- 1 cup onion, finely chopped
- 2 cloves garlic, sliced
- 1 (14-ounce) can diced tomatoes, with juice
- ½ teaspoon black pepper
- 1½ teaspoons seasoned salt
- 1 cup green cabbage, finely chopped
- 1 (5-ounce) can smoked ground ham

Directions:
1. Wash navy beans according to package directions.
2. In a large saucepan, heat 1-quart water to boiling. Remove from heat; add beans, cover and let sit for one hour to soften; drain.
3. Add broth, water, carrots, onion, garlic, tomatoes, pepper, seasoned salt, cabbage, and ham. Cover; cook on low heat for 3-4 hours, or until beans become very soft. Stir occasionally.
4. Using a potato masher, mash beans until about half of them are broken apart; stir to blend.

Macros per Serving & Nutrition Facts
- Calories 177
- Total Fat 2g
- Total Carbohydrate 26g
- Protein 14g

French Onion Soup

French onion soup has such great flavor yet has only a few ingredients. This soup is wonderfully easy to throw together for a quick lunch.

Serves: 6
Overall time 40 minutes

Ingredients:
- 1 tablespoon olive oil
- 2 cups sweet onions, finely chopped
- 4 cups chicken broth
- ½ cup dry red wine
- 1 teaspoon garlic, finely chopped
- 6 slices French bread, 1-inch thick
- 6 tablespoons Parmesan cheese, freshly grated

Directions:
1. In a large saucepan, add olive oil and onions; cook over medium heat, stirring often, until onions are browned.
2. Add broth, wine, and garlic; cover and cook over low heat for 25 minutes.
3. Meanwhile, toast bread until lightly browned; place one piece of toast in bottom of individual soup bowls; sprinkle each toast with 1 tablespoon Parmesan cheese.
4. Pour soup over toast to serve.

Macros per Serving & Nutrition Facts
- Calories 190
- Total Fat 9g
- Total Carbohydrate 21g
- Protein 7g

-

Cheesy Cauliflower Soup

My father doesn't like vegetables, but he always asks for seconds of this soup. Use homemade chicken broth whenever possible as it gives a richer flavor.

Serves: 6-8
Overall time 45 minutes

Ingredients:
- 3 tablespoons olive oil
- ¾ cup onions, finely chopped
- 5 cups chicken broth
- 1 cup water
- 1 medium cauliflower, cut into florets
- ⅛ teaspoon rosemary
- ⅛ teaspoon thyme
- ¼ teaspoon black pepper
- 2 tablespoons butter, melted
- ¼ cup whole flour
- 2 cups cheddar cheese, shredded

Directions:
1. In a large saucepan, heat oil; add onions and cook over medium heat until softened, about 5 minutes.
2. Add broth, water, cauliflower, rosemary, thyme, and pepper. Cover; cook over low heat for 30 minutes, or until cauliflower is tender. Remove from heat.
3. Using a potato masher, mash cauliflower mixture until cauliflower is broken into small pieces; return to heat.
4. In a small bowl, combine melted butter and flour; mix well, then add to soup, cooking over low heat and stirring until soup is thickened to desired consistency.
5. Add cheese, one cup at a time, stirring until cheese is melted. Serve.

Macros per Serving & Nutrition Facts
- Calories 252
- Total Fat 14g
- Total Carbohydrate 24g
- Protein 0g

Creamy Chicken Vegetable Soup

This recipe was given to me by a dental assistant—she often made this soup for her in-laws when they began needing soft foods. They loved it, and so will you!

Serves: 6
Overall time 1 hour 45 minutes

Ingredients:
- 2 tablespoons olive oil
- ½ cup onions, finely chopped
- ½ cup carrots, thinly sliced or shredded
- ½ cup potatoes, diced
- ½ cup green beans
- ½ cup peas
- 1 cup chicken, finely chopped
- 1 (14-ounce) can chicken broth
- ¼ teaspoon black pepper
- 1¼ cups milk
- 1 (10¾-ounce) can cream of celery soup
- 1 (10¾-ounce) can cream of cheddar cheese soup

Directions:
1. In a large saucepan, heat oil; add onions and carrots; cook and stir until softened, about 5 minutes.
2. Add potatoes, green beans, peas, chicken, broth, and pepper. Cover, and cook over low heat for 1½ hours, or until vegetables are soft; stir occasionally.

3. Add milk, celery soup and cheddar cheese soup; stir and continue cooking until heated throughout.

Macros per Serving & Nutrition Facts
- Calories 125
- Total Fat 3.6g
- Total Carbohydrate 15.6g
- Protein 7.6g

Clam Chowder

When choosing turkey bacon be sure to use mild, or unflavored, turkey bacon. A strong turkey bacon, such as hickory smoked, can overpower the taste of the clam chowder.

Serves: 6
Overall time 45 minutes

Ingredients:
- 1 cup onion, finely chopped
- 3 cups potatoes, diced
- 1 clove garlic, finely chopped
- 2 slices turkey bacon, cooked and finely crumbled
- 1 teaspoon salt
- ¼ teaspoon black pepper
- 1 (8-ounce) bottle clam juice
- 2 (7-ounce) cans minced clams
- 3 tablespoons whole flour
- 1 cup milk
- 2 cups half-and-half

Directions:
1. Remove starch from potatoes by slicing them and soaking in lukewarm water and straining 4 times.

2. In a large saucepan, combine onion, potatoes, garlic, turkey bacon, salt, pepper, and clam juice; cover and cook on low for 30 minutes, or until vegetables are soft.
3. In a small bowl, stir flour into milk; mix well.
4. Add flour and milk mixture to saucepan along with half-and-half and clams with their liquid; stirring constantly, cook over medium heat until chowder thickens to desired consistency.
5. Transfer the mixture to a blender; blend until smooth and return to saucepan.

Macros per Serving & Nutrition Facts
- Calories 163
- Total Fat 5.83g
- Total Carbohydrate 19.01g
- Protein 8.83g

Cream of Broccoli Soup

If you love broccoli, this is the soup for you. Blended smooth, it goes down easy, is flavorful, and goes great with your favorite sandwich.

Serves: 6
Overall time 45 minutes

Ingredients:
- 4 cups broccoli florets
- 1 cup onion, chopped
- 1 tablespoon celery flakes
- 1 clove garlic, chopped
- 1 medium potato, peeled and diced
- 1 (14-ounce) chicken broth
- 2 cups milk
- 1½ cups cheddar cheese, shredded
- ¼ teaspoon thyme
- ½ teaspoon salt
- ¼ teaspoon white pepper

Directions:
1. In a medium saucepan, add broccoli, onion, celery flakes, garlic, potato, and chicken broth; bring to near boiling; reduce heat, cover and cook over low heat for 30 minutes, or until vegetables are soft.
2. Transfer cooked vegetables with broth to a blender; blend until smooth.
3. Return blended vegetables to saucepan; add milk, cheese, thyme, salt, and pepper.
4. Continue cooking over low heat until cheese is melted, stirring constantly.

Macros per Serving & Nutrition Facts
- Calories 150
- Total Fat 7g
- Total Carbohydrate 15g
- Protein 5g

Chicken Noodle Soup

Using home cooked chicken with homemade broth will add depth of flavor to this soup. Even if you only have one cup of homemade broth to add along with canned broth it will help create that homemade flavor for this lovely "comfort" soup.

Serves: 6-8
Overall time 1 hour 30 minutes

Ingredients:
- 1 tablespoon olive or canola oil
- ¾ cup onion, finely chopped
- ⅔ cup carrots, shredded
- 4 cups chicken broth
- 2 cups water

- 1 tablespoon dried celery flakes
- 1 bay leaf
- 1 cup cooked chicken, finely chopped
- 1 tablespoon parsley flakes
- 1 teaspoon seasoned salt
- ¼ teaspoon black pepper, or to taste
- 1½ cups egg noodles, uncooked and broken into 3-inch pieces

Directions:
1. In a large saucepan, add oil, carrots and onion then allow to cook on medium heat until soft, about 5 minutes.
2. Add broth, water, celery flakes, bay leaf, and chicken; cover and cook over low heat for 1 hour, stirring occasionally.
3. Stir in parsley, seasoned salt, pepper, and noodles; cover and continue cooking over low heat for 25 minutes. Remove bay leaf before serving.

Macros per Serving & Nutrition Facts
- Calories 220
- Total Fat 5g
- Total Carbohydrate 24g
- Protein 18g

Cream of Potato Soup

This wonderfully versatile recipe can be easily changed to accommodate your tastes. It can be enjoyed as a simple potato soup, or other ingredients can be added, such as ham, cheese, or vegetables. For a smoother soup, just put it in a blender to puree or mash lightly.

Serves: 6
Overall time 45 minutes

Ingredients:
- 1 tablespoon butter
- 1 cup onion, finely chopped
- 3 cups diced potatoes
- 3 cups chicken broth
- ¼ teaspoon black pepper
- ½ teaspoon salt
- ½ teaspoon garlic powder
- ¼ cup whole flour
- 1½ cups milk
- 1 cup sharp cheddar cheese, shredded (optional)

Directions:
1. In a medium saucepan, melt butter over medium heat. Add onion; stir and cook until onions are softened.
2. Add potatoes, chicken broth, pepper, salt, and garlic powder, plus ham if desired.
3. Cover; cook over low heat until potatoes are tender and easily fall apart, about 40 minutes.
4. In a small bowl, combine flour and milk; mix until smooth. Stir flour mixture into soup; continue cooking and stirring until soup is thickened and of desired consistency.
5. Add cheese if desired; stir just until melted and smooth. Serve.

Macros per Serving & Nutrition Facts
- Calories 225.7
- Total Fat 5.7g
- Total Carbohydrate 39g
- Protein 4.6g

Chicken and Bean Soup

This soup was love at first bite for me. It's one to make over and over again. I usually use veggie bacon in place of regular bacon as it becomes soft in soup.

Serves: 2-4
Overall time 40 minutes
Ingredients:
- 1 tablespoon olive oil
- ½ cup onion, finely chopped
- 1 clove garlic, finely chopped
- 1 (14½-ounce) can chicken broth, with roasted vegetable and herb flavoring
- ½ cup water
- 1 cup canned great northern beans, rinsed and drained
- ¾ cup chicken, cooked and finely chopped
- ¼ teaspoon black pepper
- 1 strip veggie bacon, cooked and finely crumbled

Directions:
1. In a medium saucepan, heat oil; add onion and garlic, cooking over low heat until softened, about 5 minutes.
2. Add broth and water to saucepan; bring to near boiling; reduce heat.
3. Add remaining ingredients; cover and cook over low heat for 30 minutes. Stir occasionally.

Macros per Serving & Nutrition Facts
- Calories 225.7
- Total Fat 5.7g
- Total Carbohydrate 39g
- Protein 4.6g

Slow Cooker Recipes

Almost Lasagna

This is a quick and easy lasagna-like dish for the lasagna lovers in the crowd.

Serves: 8
Overall time 5-6 hours

Ingredients:
- 1 (8-ounce) package bowtie pasta
- 1½ pounds lean ground chicken
- 1 medium onion, finely chopped
- 1 (26-ounce) jar pasta sauce
- 1½ cups small-curd cottage cheese
- 1 (16-ounce) package Mozzarella cheese, shredded

Directions:
1. Cook pasta according to package directions; drain.
2. Meanwhile, in a large skillet, cook ground chicken and onion, stirring until ground chicken is browned and crumbly and onions are softened. Drain fat.
3. Add pasta sauce to ground chicken; stir well.
4. Place half of the ground chicken mixture in the slow cooker; then add a half of the pasta on top followed by a half of the cottage cheese then half of the Mozzarella cheese.
5. Repeat the layers with the remaining half of the chicken, pasta, cottage cheese, then Mozzarella cheese.
6. Cover; cook on Low 5-6 hours.

Macros per Serving & Nutrition Facts
- Calories 212
- Total Fat 7 g
- Total Carbohydrate 5 g
- Protein 18 g

Apple Sauerkraut with Chicken Sausage

Such a simple yet tasty dish to make, this one goes well with noodles or mashed potatoes. For easier chewing, be sure to finely chop the sauerkraut before adding to slow cooker.

Serves: 4
Overall time 6 hours

Ingredients:
- 1 (14-ounce) can sauerkraut, finely chopped
- 1-pound smoked Chicken sausage, skinless
- 2 cooking apples, peeled and sliced
- ¼ cup stevia
- ½ cup apple cider or apple juice

Directions:
1. Place half of the sauerkraut in the bottom of a slow cooker.
2. Spread half of the apple slices over the sauerkraut, then sprinkle with half of the stevia.
3. Cut the chicken sausage into 1-inch pieces; add to slow cooker.
4. Place the remaining apple slices on top of the chicken sausage, sprinkle apples with remaining stevia, then top with the remaining sauerkraut.
5. Pour the apple cider, or juice, over all.
6. Cover; cook on Low for 6 hours.

Macros per Serving & Nutrition Facts
- Calories 284
- Total Fat 32.9 g
- Total Carbohydrate 30.5 g
- Protein 16.3 g

Barbeque Chicken and Beans

Eating this dish with corn bread on the side is a simple yet satisfying meal. This dish uses veggie bacon, because it becomes soft while cooking, however, you can use finely crumbled regular bacon if that is soft enough for you after it cooks in a sauce.

Serves: 8
Overall time 3 hours 30 minutes

Ingredients:
- ½ pound ground chicken
- ⅓ cup onion, finely chopped
- 2 slices veggie bacon, crisp, crumbled
- Great Northern beans (15oz., canned)
- 1 (15oz) can pinto beans
- 1 (15oz) can pork and beans
- ½ cup barbeque sauce
- ¼ cup green pepper, finely chopped (optional)

Directions:
1. In a medium skillet, cook ground chicken and onion, stirring until ground chicken is browned and crumbly and onions are softened. Drain fat.
2. In a slow cooker, add all ingredients; mix well.
3. Cover; cook on High heat for 3½ hours, or until onions are of desired softness.

Macros per Serving & Nutrition Facts
- Calories 158
- Total Fat 4 g
- Total Carbohydrate 7 g
- Protein 10 g

Saucy Chopped Steaks

So tender and delicious. Any type of chopped steak can be used in this recipe. Serve these soft steaks with your favorite soft side dish.

Serves: 4
Overall time 8 hours

Ingredients:
- 1 (10¾-ounce) can cream of mushroom soup
- 4 chopped steaks
- 1 large onion, chopped
- 2 carrots, peeled, cut into 1-inch slices

Directions:
1. Place half of the soup into slow cooker; spread evenly across bottom.
2. Place steaks side-by-side in slow cooker; spoon remaining soup evenly over top of steaks.
3. Place onions and carrots on top.
4. Cook on Low for 8 hours, or until tender.

Macros per Serving & Nutrition Facts
- Calories 56
- Total Fat 2.9 g
- Total Carbohydrate 7.1 g
- Protein 1.2 g

Chicken Patty Stew

The addition of red wine gives this stew a depth of flavor you will appreciate.

Serves: 4
Overall time 6 hours

Ingredients:
- 1-pound ground chicken
- 1 large tomato, peeled and diced
- 2 carrots, sliced
- 2 medium onions, sliced
- ¼ pound fresh mushrooms, sliced
- 1 tablespoon dried celery flakes
- 3 medium potatoes, peeled, quartered
- 1 clove garlic, minced
- 1 cup chicken broth
- ½ cup red wine
- 1 teaspoon salt
- ¼ teaspoon black pepper
- 3 tablespoons cornstarch

Directions:
1. Form chicken into four patties; place side by side in a large skillet, brown both sides.
2. Place patties in a slow cooker; top with tomato, carrots, onions, mushrooms, celery flakes and potatoes.
3. In a small bowl, combine garlic, chicken broth, wine, salt and pepper; mix well.
4. In a separate bowl, mix cornstarch with a few tablespoons of broth mixture; add cornstarch mixture to the broth mixture, stir to combine.
5. Pour broth mixture into slow cooker over chicken and vegetables; cook on Low for 6 hours, or until vegetables are tender.

Macros per Serving & Nutrition Facts
- Calories 246
- Total Fat 11.4 g
- Total Carbohydrate 9 g
- Protein 16 g

Chicken Filled Rigatoni

This dish has few ingredients, is simple to make, and yet is full of flavor.

Serves: 8-10
Overall time 4-5 hours

Ingredients:
- 1 (12-ounce) package of rigatoni pasta
- 1½ pounds of lean ground chicken
- 1½ cups onions, finely chopped
- 1 (20-ounce) jar pasta sauce
- 3 cups Mozzarella cheese, shredded
- 1 cup fresh mushrooms, finely chopped

Directions:
1. Cook rigatoni according to package directions; drain.
2. Meanwhile, in a medium skillet, cook ground chicken and onions, stirring until ground chicken is browned and crumbly and onions are softened. Drain fat.
3. Place half of the pasta sauce in the slow cooker; add a half of your ground chicken mixture on top followed by a half of the rigatoni, half of the cheese, and half of the mushrooms.
4. Layer remaining ingredients in same order as Step 3.
5. Cover; cook on Low 4–5 hours.

Macros per Serving & Nutrition Facts
- Calories 189
- Total Fat 8.5 g
- Total Carbohydrate 7 g
- Protein 27 g

Chicken Cacciatore

Chicken Cacciatore is delicious served over hot linguini noodles or spaghetti noodles. For even easier chewing, remove cooked chicken, debone, cut into small pieces, then mix chicken pieces back into slow cooker before serving.

Serves: 6
Overall time 6-7 hours

Ingredients:
- 2½ pounds chicken legs and thighs
- 2 medium onions, finely chopped
- 2 medium green peppers, chopped
- 1 bay leaf
- 2 cloves garlic, sliced
- 1 (16-ounce) can stewed tomatoes
- 1 (8-ounce) can tomato sauce
- ½ teaspoon salt
- ¼ teaspoon black pepper
- ½ teaspoon oregano
- ½ teaspoon basil
- ¼ cup white wine (optional)

Directions:
1. Place chicken in bottom of slow cooker.
2. Place onions, green peppers, and bay leaf on top of chicken
3. In a medium bowl, combine garlic, tomatoes, tomato sauce, salt, pepper, oregano and basil, plus wine if desired; mix well.
4. Pour tomato mixture over vegetables and chicken.
5. Cover; cook on Low 6–7 hours, or until tender. Remove bay leaf before serving.
6. If needed, remove cooked chicken, debone, and cut into small pieces; mix chicken pieces back into slow cooker.

Macros per Serving & Nutrition Facts
- Calories 335
- Total Fat 12.8 g
- Total Carbohydrate 6.5 g
- Protein 7.2 g

Chicken Stew

This stew comes out just right – the sauce is not too thick, not too thin. If you prefer dark meat, simply substitute chicken thighs for the breasts.

Serves: 4-6
Overall time 7-8 hours

Ingredients:
- 1½ cups water
- 1 cup chicken broth
- 2 (.87- ounce) packages chicken gravy mix
- 2 cloves garlic, finely chopped
- 1 tablespoon parsley
- ½ teaspoon black pepper
- 5 carrots, peeled, cut into 1-inch slices
- 1½ cups green beans, frozen or fresh
- 4 boneless chicken breasts (1½ pounds)
- 3 tablespoon whole flour
- ⅓ cup water
- 1 (6.3-ounce) tube refrigerated buttermilk biscuits

Directions:
1. Combine 1½ cups water, broth, gravy mix, garlic, parsley, and pepper in slow cooker; mix well. Add carrots, green beans, and chicken.
2. Cover, and cook on Low for 7-8 hours, or until tender.
3. Remove cooked chicken and cut into small pieces; set aside.

4. In a small bowl, combine flour and ⅓ cup water; stir into slow cooker.
5. Mix in chicken pieces; cover, set control on High and cook one more hour.
6. Meanwhile, bake biscuits according to package directions; serve chicken stew on top of halved biscuits.

Macros per Serving & Nutrition Facts
- Calories 117
- Total Fat 3.9 g
- Total Carbohydrate 9.9 g
- Protein 10.2 g

Chicken Tetrazzini

If you prefer dark meat, just substitute boneless chicken thighs for the breasts in this recipe.

Serves: 6
Overall time 5 hours

Ingredients:
- 1¼ pounds chicken breast tenderloins
- 1 cup chicken broth
- ½ cup white wine
- 1 medium onion, finely chopped
- ¼ teaspoon dried thyme
- 1 teaspoon salt
- ½ teaspoon black pepper
- 2½ tablespoons cornstarch
- ¼ cup water
- 1 cup fresh mushrooms, finely chopped
- ½ cup half-and-half or whole milk
- ½ pound spaghetti, broken into 3-inch pieces
- ½ cup Parmesan cheese, grated

Directions:
1. Add chicken to slow cooker.
2. In a medium bowl, combine broth, wine, onion, thyme, salt and pepper; pour over chicken.
3. Cover; cook on Low for 5 hours, or until chicken is tender; break chicken into bite sized pieces.
4. In a small bowl, combine cornstarch and water; stir until smooth. Add cornstarch mixture to slow cooker; stir and add mushrooms; cover; cook on High for 20 minutes. 5. Meanwhile, cook spaghetti according to package; drain.
5. Stir half-and-half, spaghetti, and cheese into slow cooker. Cover; cook on High another 5 minutes, or until heated throughout.

Macros per Serving & Nutrition Facts
- Calories 299
- Total Fat 9.8 g
- Total Carbohydrate 20.5 g
- Protein 32.6 g

Scalloped Potatoes and Ham

This dish should be called "impossible scalloped potatoes" as it has little liquid yet turns out soft and tasty.

Serves: 6-8
Overall time 7-8 hours

Ingredients:
- 2 (6-ounce) cans ground smoked ham
- 8 medium potatoes, thinly sliced
- 2 small onions, finely chopped
- ¼ teaspoon black pepper
- 1 cup Cheddar cheese, shredded

- 1 (10¾-ounce) can cream of mushroom soup
- ⅔ soup can milk

Directions:

1. Remove starch from potatoes by slicing them and soaking in lukewarm water and straining 4 times.
2. In a small bowl, break the ham into small pieces.
3. Place half of the ham, potatoes, and onions into slow cooker; sprinkle the cheese and pepper over the top.
4. Layer the remaining ham, potatoes, and onions into slow cooker.
5. In a medium bowl, combine soup with milk; pour soup mixture into the slow cooker evenly over the top of the potato mixture.
6. Cover; cook on Low for 7-8 hours, or until tender.

Macros per Serving & Nutrition Facts

- Calories 358
- Total Fat 4.7 g
- Total Carbohydrate 18 g
- Protein 9.9 g

Chicken with Broccoli and Quinoa

This dish is quick and easy to make. It can be put together the night before and kept in the refrigerator until ready to cook the next day.

Serves: 4-6
Overall time 3 hours

Ingredients:

- 2 tablespoons vegetable oil
- 1 medium onion, finely chopped
- 1 clove garlic, finely chopped
- 3 cups fresh or frozen broccoli florets, chopped
- 2 cups cooked chicken, finely chopped

- 1 (10¾-ounce) can cream of chicken soup
- 1 (12-ounce) can evaporated milk
- 3 cups white quinoa, cooked
- 1½ cups Cheddar cheese, shredded
- ½ teaspoon black pepper
- ½ cup fresh mushrooms, finely chopped

Directions:
1. In a large skillet, heat the oil over medium heat; add the onion, garlic, and broccoli, cooking and stirring until softened, about 5 minutes.
2. In a large bowl, combine broccoli mixture, chicken, soup, evaporated milk, quinoa, cheese, pepper, and mushrooms; mix well.
3. Pour into slow cooker.
4. Cover; cook on Low for 3 hours.

Macros per Serving & Nutrition Facts
- Calories 354
- Total Fat 22.9 g
- Total Carbohydrate 15.8 g
- Protein 20.7 g

Creamy Chicken and Noodles

The chicken comes out so tender. However, if you need extra softness, when the chicken is cooked remove the chicken from the slow cooker and take the meat off the bones. Finely chop the chicken then stir back into the slow cooker.

Serves: 4-6
Overall time 8 hours

Ingredients:
- 2 (10¾-ounce) cans cream of chicken soup
- 1½-2 pounds chicken legs and thighs

- 2 cups carrots, peeled and sliced
- 1½ cups onion, chopped
- 1 cup peas, frozen or fresh
- 1 bay leaf
- 1 tablespoon parsley
- ½ cup water
- 1 teaspoon thyme
- ¼ teaspoon black pepper
- 1 (8-ounce) package noodles

Directions:
1. Spread one can of soup around your slow cooker; add chicken pieces side by side on top of soup.
2. Place carrots, onions, peas, and bay leaf on top of chicken.
3. In a bowl, combine remaining soup, parsley, water, thyme, and pepper; pour into slow cooker over chicken and vegetables.
4. Cover; cook for about 8 hours on low, or until tender.
5. Cook noodles according to package directions; drain.
6. Spoon chicken and vegetables over noodles to serve.

Macros per Serving & Nutrition Facts
- Calories 291
- Total Fat 13.6 g
- Total Carbohydrate 10.5 g
- Protein 30.8 g

Creamy Pork Chop

This is a wonderfully quick and easy dish to put together, and the pork chops come out so tender you can cut them with your fork. For extra softness, remove the cooked pork chops from the slow cooker, take the meat off the bones, finely chop the meat, then stir back into the slow cooker.

Serves: 6
Overall time 8-9 hours

Ingredients:
- 6 pork chops
- 1 (14¾-ounce) can cream of chicken soup
- ½ teaspoon garlic powder
- 1½ teaspoons dry mustard

Directions:
1. Spread half of soup evenly across bottom of slow cooker.
2. Place pork chops side by side on top of soup.
3. In a medium bowl, combine remaining soup, garlic, and mustard. Spread over pork chops.
4. Cover; cook on Low 8-9 hours, or under tender.

Macros per Serving & Nutrition Facts
- Calories 377
- Total Fat 20.4 g
- Total Carbohydrate 4 g
- Protein 41.7 g

Cold Snacks Recipes

Mozzarella and Tomato Salad V 20

Simple and fresh – my favorite kind of side dish! This one can also be used as a lovely appetizer.

Serves: 6
Overall time 15 minutes

Ingredients:
- 6 ounces fresh Mozzarella cheese, cut into ¼-inch slices
- 4 medium tomatoes, peeled and sliced
- ¼ cup fresh basil leaves, finely chopped
- ⅓ cup olive oil
- 2 tablespoons white wine vinegar
- ½ teaspoon sugar
- salt and pepper to taste

Directions:
1. In a medium sized shallow serving dish, layer Mozzarella, tomatoes, and basil.
2. In a small bowl, add oil, vinegar, sugar, salt, and pepper; whisk to combine.
3. Pour oil mixture over Mozzarella and tomatoes; cover, refrigerate to chill.

Macros per Serving & Nutrition Facts
- Calories 132
- Total Fat 7.4g
- Total Carbohydrate 11.9 g
- Protein 8g

Potato Salad V

A traditional summer side dish, I usually put several hard-boiled eggs in it as my parents sometimes eat a small dish of potato salad as a simple lunch. I use veggie bacon because it becomes soft in salad dressing while still giving that lovely bacon taste.

Serves: 6-8
Overall time 30 minutes

Ingredients:
- 4 medium potatoes, cooked, peeled, and diced
- 4 hard cooked eggs, peeled and chopped
- 2 pieces veggie bacon, crisp cooked and crumbled
- 1 teaspoon onion powder
- ½ cup mayonnaise
- ¼ cup Ranch dressing
- 1½ teaspoons vinegar
- 2 teaspoons sugar
- 1 teaspoon prepared mustard
- 1 tablespoon chives
- 1 tablespoon Parmesan cheese, grated
- ½ teaspoon seasoned salt
- ¼ teaspoon black pepper

Directions:
1. In a large bowl, place cooled diced potatoes, chopped eggs, and veggie bacon crumbles.
2. In a medium bowl, add mayonnaise, Ranch dressing, vinegar, sugar, chives, Parmesan cheese, seasoned salt and pepper; stir until well blended.
3. Pour mayonnaise dressing mixture over potato mixture; stir gently to combine; cover, refrigerate.

Macros per Serving & Nutrition Facts
- Calories 197
- Total Fat 11 g
- Total Carbohydrate 18.9 g
- Protein 5.8 g

Cauliflower Pasta Salad V 20

Tri-color pasta allows this simple pasta salad to make a lovely presentation. If you don't have tri-color pasta available, you can add color to this dish by adding a cup of tender green peas or diced tomatoes.

Serves: 8
Overall time 15 minutes

Ingredients:
- 2 cups cauliflower florets (about 1 small head)
- 1 (8-ounce) package tri-color rotini or bowtie pasta
- ¼ cup red onion, finely chopped, or ½ teaspoon onion powder
- ¼ cup Parmesan cheese, grated
- ½ cup Italian salad dressing

Directions:
1. In a medium saucepan, cook the cauliflower in hot water until soft; drain and refrigerate to cool.
2. Meanwhile, in a medium saucepan, cook pasta according to package directions; drain and refrigerate to cool.
3. Cut cauliflower into bite-size pieces, cutting off any tough stalks.
4. In a large bowl, place cooled cauliflower, pasta, onion and Parmesan cheese.
5. Pour salad dressing over cauliflower mixture; toss gently to combine.
6. Cover; refrigerate to chill.

Macros per Serving & Nutrition Facts
- Calories 57
- Total Fat 4.1 g
- Total Carbohydrate 3.9 g
- Protein 1.5 g

Pea Salad V 20

The red onion, dill, and fresh lemon juice combine to make this salad flavorsome. Remember, if even finely chopped onion is problematic for you, replace the onion with a half teaspoon or so of onion powder.

Serves: 4-6
Overall time 15 minutes

Ingredients:
- 1 (16-ounce) package frozen peas
- ¼ cup red onion, finely chopped
- 1 cup cheddar cheese, shredded
- 3 hard cooked eggs, finely chopped
- ½ cup mayonnaise
- ¼ cup sour cream
- 1 tablespoon lemon juice
- 1½ teaspoons dill weed
- ½ teaspoon salt
- ½ teaspoon black pepper

Directions:
1. Cook peas according to package directions, or until tender; drain; refrigerate to chill.
2. In a large bowl, combine chilled peas, onion, cheese, and eggs.
3. In a small bowl, whisk together mayonnaise, sour cream, lemon juice, dill, salt and pepper.
4. Pour mayonnaise mixture over pea mixture; stir gently to combine.
5. Cover; refrigerate to chill.

Macros per Serving & Nutrition Facts
- Calories 167

- Total Fat 12.4 g
- Total Carbohydrate 6.3 g
- Protein 7.5 g

Cooked Carrot Salad V 20

This salad is so incredibly simple, and yet so enjoyable. Use any of the various Ranch dressing flavors available or substitute your favorite salad dressing.

Serves: 4-6
Overall time 15 minutes

Ingredients:
- 2 cups water
- 1 tablespoon sugar
- 1 bunch of carrots
- 3 tablespoons Ranch dressing

Directions:
1. Peel carrots and cut each carrot into thirds, crossways.
2. In a medium saucepan, bring water and sugar to a boil; add carrots. Cover; cook over low heat until carrots are soft, about 20-30 minutes.
3. Drain; cover and refrigerate to chill.
4. Cut cooled carrots into 1-inch pieces and place in a serving dish.
5. Drizzle salad dressing over carrots, serve.

Macros per Serving & Nutrition Facts
- Calories 150
- Total Fat 2g
- Total Carbohydrate 16 g
- Protein 5g

Creamy Cucumber Salad V 20

Sliced very thin, and eaten in small bites, this dish should be soft enough for most cucumber lovers to be able to enjoy the taste of summer. You can also chop cucumber slices into smaller pieces for easier chewing. Refrigerating overnight before serving adds to the softness.

Serves: 8
Overall time 15 minutes

Ingredients:
- 3 medium cucumbers
- 1 tablespoon sugar
- ½ cup sour cream
- 1½ teaspoons salt
- ½ teaspoon onion powder
- 1 tablespoon white vinegar

Directions:
1. Peel cucumbers; cut in half lengthwise, then slice very thin; set aside.
2. In a medium bowl, combine sugar, sour cream, salt, onion powder, and vinegar.
3. Add cucumber slices to bowl; stir until cucumbers are well coated with dressing; refrigerate for several hours to chill and soften.

Macros per Serving & Nutrition Facts
- Calories 48.6
- Total Fat 3.2g
- Total Carbohydrate 4.5g
- Protein 1.4g

Marinated Tomato Slices V

A pretty looking dish, this is a simple way to enjoy the fruits of summer. Eat this with bread or rolls, if you like, so you can soak up the tasty sauce.

Serves: 8-10
Overall time 3 hours

Ingredients:
- 4 large tomatoes
- ¼ cup olive oil
- 1 tablespoon lemon juice
- 1 teaspoon sugar
- ½ teaspoon salt
- ½ teaspoon oregano
- 1 tablespoon parsley

Directions:
1. Peel the tomatoes and cut into ½-inch slices; layer in an oblong shallow serving dish.
2. In a small bowl, combine oil, lemon juice, sugar, salt, oregano, and parsley mix well.
3. Pour oil mixture over tomatoes; cover and refrigerate for at least 3 hours to marinate.

Macros per Serving & Nutrition Facts
- Calories 57.3
- Total Fat 3.7g
- Total Carbohydrate 5.9g
- Protein 0.7g

Lime-Pear Gelatin V 20

Smooth and creamy, no one will guess there are healthy ingredients in this tasty side dish.

Serves: 6
Overall time 15 minutes

Ingredients:
- 1 (.3-ounce) package lime gelatin
- ¾ cup hot water
- 1 (15-ounce) can pear slices or halves, drained
- 1 (8-ounce) package cream cheese, softened

Directions:
1. In a small bowl, dissolve gelatin in hot water.
2. Place gelatin, pears, and cream cheese in a blender; blend until smooth.
3. Pour into an 8x8-inch dish; refrigerate until set.

Macros per Serving & Nutrition Facts
- Calories 12
- Total Fat 0.71g
- Total Carbohydrate 0.99g
- Protein 0.38g

Gelatin with Peaches and Cottage Cheese V 20

Our family has enjoyed this cool side dish for decades. It is especially good on a warm summer day. For an even softer gelatin dish, puree the cottage cheese and peaches before folding them into the gelatin.

Serves: 4-6
Overall time 15 minutes

Ingredients:
- 1 (.3-ounce) package cherry flavored gelatin
- 1 cup small curd cottage cheese
- 1 cup peaches, sliced or diced

Directions:
1. Prepare gelatin according to package instructions; refrigerate to chill.
2. Meanwhile, cut peach slices into bite sized pieces.
3. When gelatin is almost set, fold in cottage cheese and peaches.
4. Return to refrigerator and chill until firm.

Macros per Serving & Nutrition Facts
- Calories 220
- Total Fat 2g
- Total Carbohydrate 16g
- Protein 20g

Soft Cauliflower Salad V 20

A lovely, light soft salad. You can also substitute your favorite salad dressing for the dressing used here.

Serves: 4
Overall time 15 minutes

Ingredients:
- 4 cups water
- 3 cups cauliflower florets
- 1 bay leaf

Dressing:
- ⅓ cup olive oil
- 1 clove garlic, finely chopped

- tablespoons balsamic or white wine vinegar
- ½ teaspoon sugar
- ½ teaspoon basil
- ½ teaspoon oregano
- ⅛ teaspoon thyme or rosemary
- ⅛ teaspoon black pepper

Directions:
1. In a medium saucepan, bring 4 cups water to a boil; add cauliflower and bay leaf.
2. Cover, cook over low heat until cauliflower is soft; drain, remove bay leaf; place cauliflower in a medium bowl and refrigerate to cool.
3. Meanwhile, in a small bowl, combine olive oil, garlic, vinegar, sugar, basil, oregano, thyme, and pepper; whisk until well blended.
4. Drizzle dressing over cauliflower; toss gently to combine; cover and refrigerate to chill.

Macros per Serving & Nutrition Facts
- Calories 125
- Total Fat 6.7g
- Total Carbohydrate 14.4g
- Protein 4.9g

Homemade Applesauce V 20

I grew up with mom's homemade applesauce. You will be surprised at how easy it is to make, and how much more flavorful it is than store bought applesauce. Depending on the type of apples you use, you may need a little more or a little less water. Both Cortland and McIntosh apples make a good applesauce.

Serves: 8
Overall time 15 minutes

Ingredients:
- 8 cooking apples
- ⅓ cup water
- ⅓ cup sugar
- 1 teaspoon cinnamon (optional)

Directions:
1. Peel apples, core, and cut into quarters.
2. Place apples in a medium saucepan; add water.
3. Cover; cook on low heat until apples are very soft and mixture is thickened, about 30 minutes.
4. Mash apple mixture with a potato masher; stir in sugar, and cinnamon if desired, and continue cooking uncovered until applesauce is of desired consistency.
5. Cover; refrigerate to chill.

Macros per Serving & Nutrition Facts
- Calories 56.7
- Total Fat 0.2g
- Total Carbohydrate 14.9g
- Protein 0.1g

Hot Snacks Recipes

Broccoli and Pasta V

You can use noodles or any pasta of your choice for this colorful Italian dish.

Serves: 4
Overall time 35 minutes

Ingredients:
- 1 (8-ounce) package wheat noodles
- 2 tablespoons olive oil
- 2 tablespoons green onion, finely chopped
- 2 cups broccoli florets, finely chopped
- 1 (14-ounce) can diced tomatoes, undrained
- ½ teaspoon oregano
- ½ teaspoon thyme
- ½ teaspoon black pepper
- 2 tablespoons Parmesan cheese, grated

Directions:
1. Cook noodles according to package directions; drain.
2. Meanwhile, in a medium skillet, add oil and onion; cook over medium heat until onion is softened, about 5 minutes.
3. Add broccoli, tomatoes with their juice, oregano, thyme, and pepper; stir.
4. Cover; cook over low heat until broccoli is tender, about 20 minutes.
5. Stir in cooked noodles; continue cooking until heated throughout; top with Parmesan cheese before serving.

Macros per Serving & Nutrition Facts
- Calories 275
- Total Fat 6.9g
- Total Carbohydrate 16g
- Protein 13.6g

Gnocchi in Cream Sauce V 20

You can enjoy this recipe as a simple side dish or create a more colorful, dashing dish by adding soft vegetables to the sauce, such as chopped olives, diced tomatoes, cooked peas, or finely chopped spinach.

Serves: 4
Overall time 10 minutes

Ingredients:
- 1 (12-ounce) package potato gnocchi
- ⅔ cup half-and-half
- 2 ounces cream cheese, diced
- ½ teaspoon salt
- ½ teaspoon garlic powder
- ¼ teaspoon oregano
- ¼ teaspoon basil
- ¼ teaspoon black pepper

Directions:
1. Cook gnocchi according to package directions; drain.
2. Meanwhile, in a saucepan add half-and-half, cream cheese, salt, garlic powder, oregano, basil and pepper; cook over medium heat until heated throughout and cream cheese is melted, about 10 minutes.
3. Add ½ cup cooked soft vegetable, if desired.
4. Place cooked gnocchi in serving dish; pour cream sauce over gnocchi.

Macros per Serving & Nutrition Facts
- Calories 361.7
- Total Fat 10.9g
- Total Carbohydrate 56.8g
- Protein 9.5g

Apple Noodles V

The recipe for this delightfully different side dish can easily be doubled to serve a group, such as for brunch or to take to a potluck dinner.

Serves: 6
Overall time 30 minutes

Ingredients:
- 1 (8-ounce) package noodles
- 2 tablespoons butter
- 2 eggs, lightly beaten
- ¼ cup sugar
- ½ cup sour cream
- 1 cup small-curd cottage cheese
- ¼ cup milk
- ½ teaspoon vanilla
- 1 medium to large cooking apple, shredded
- 1 teaspoon cinnamon sugar (optional)

Directions:
1. Cook noodles according to package instructions.
2. Transfer drained noodles to large bowl; add butter to noodles; stirring until butter is melted and noodles are coated.
3. Add eggs, sugar, sour cream, cottage cheese, milk, vanilla and apple; mix well.
4. Pour mixture into a greased 8x8-inch baking dish.
5. Sprinkle with cinnamon sugar if desired.
6. Cover; bake in a 350-degree oven for 30 minutes, or until set.

Macros per Serving & Nutrition Facts
- Calories 191
- Total Fat 14.3g
- Total Carbohydrate 16.5g
- Protein 0.4g

Fettuccine Alfredo V 20

This side dish is a little on the rich side due to the cream and butter, but if you don't need to worry about calories – or need to add calories to your diet – this is a side dish that is so tasty and so simple to make, you can't go wrong.

Serves: 4
Overall time 10 minutes

Ingredients:
- 6-ounces zoodles, uncooked
- ½ cup light cream
- 1 tablespoon butter
- ½ cup fresh Parmesan cheese, grated
- black pepper

Directions:
1. Add zoodles to a heated saucepan over medium heat.
2. Add light cream, butter and Parmesan cheese; stir until butter is melted and fettuccine is well coated.
3. Sprinkle with black pepper; serve.

Macros per Serving & Nutrition Facts
- Calories 520
- Total Fat 12g
- Total Carbohydrate 23g
- Protein 16g

Baked Acorn Squash V

This dish is so tender, so tasty, so easy to make, and looks pretty, too – the best of all worlds.

Serves: 4
Overall time 1 hour
Ingredients:
- 2 acorn squash
- 4 teaspoons butter
- 4 tablespoons maple syrup

Directions:
1. Cut each squash in half lengthwise; remove seeds and any fibrous material.
2. In a 9x13-inch baking dish, place squash halves side by side, with cut side up.
3. Place 1 teaspoon butter and 1 tablespoon maple syrup into each half.
4. Bake at 350 degrees for 1 hour, or until soft.

Macros per Serving & Nutrition Facts
- Calories 115
- Total Fat 0.3g
- Total Carbohydrate 23g
- Protein 2.3g

Creamed Spinach V 20

This is a traditional recipe for creamed spinach—the kind you remember from days gone by.

Serves: 8
Overall time 10 minutes

Ingredients:
- (10-ounce) packages frozen spinach, thawed, finely
- chopped
- 2 tablespoons butter
- 1 small clove garlic, finely chopped

- 2 tablespoons onion, finely chopped

Sauce:
- tablespoons butter
- 2 tablespoons whole flour
- 1 cup milk
- ¼ teaspoon salt
- ⅛ teaspoon black pepper
- ⅛ teaspoon nutmeg

Directions:
1. Cook spinach according to package directions.
2. Meanwhile, in a small skillet, melt butter over medium heat; add onion and garlic; stir and cook until softened, about 5 minutes. Add spinach; stir gently to combine and transfer to a serving bowl.
3. Meanwhile, in a small saucepan, melt butter over low heat; add flour, milk, salt, pepper, and nutmeg; stir until thickened to desired consistency.
4. Pour sauce over spinach; stir to combine. Serve.

Macros per Serving & Nutrition Facts
- Calories 148
- Total Fat 9.02g
- Total Carbohydrate 11.94g
- Protein 6.66g

Carrot Patties V 20

Try adding a dollop of warmed applesauce on top before serving for even more flavor and softness.

Serves: 4
Overall time 10 minutes

Ingredients:

- 2 eggs, lightly beaten
- 3 cups carrots, cooked, mashed, and any fibrous pieces
- removed
- 3 tablespoons butter, melted
- ⅓ cup whole flour
- 2 teaspoons baking powder
- ½ cup milk
- 1 tablespoon butter

Directions:
1. In a large bowl, combine eggs, mashed carrots, butter, flour, baking powder, and milk.
2. In a large skillet, melt one-half tablespoon butter; pour one-fourth cup of batter into skillet to form each patty, flatting, if needed, to form into patties.
3. Cook on low heat about 3 minutes on each side, or until browned. Repeat step 2 for remaining batter.

Macros per Serving & Nutrition Facts
- Calories 60
- Total Fat 2g
- Total Carbohydrate 8g
- Protein 2g

Creamed Peas

For a softer dish yet, puree just before serving.

Serves: 4
Overall time 35 minutes

Ingredients:
- ⅔ cup chicken broth
- 2 cups green peas, fresh or frozen
- 2 tablespoons butter

- ⅓ cup half-and-half
- 2 tablespoons flour
- ¼ teaspoon black pepper
- ¼ teaspoon salt
- 2 tablespoons Parmesan cheese, grated (optional)

Directions:

1. In a medium saucepan, add broth and peas; bring to near boiling. Reduce heat.
2. Cover; cook on low heat 25 minutes, or until peas are tender. Add butter.
3. In a small bowl, combine half-and-half and flour; add to the peas mixture, cook and stir until thickened.
4. Add the pepper and salt, plus Parmesan cheese if desired, stirring to combine.

Macros per Serving & Nutrition Facts
- Calories 149
- Total Fat 6.2g
- Total Carbohydrate 19g
- Protein 5.9g

Cabbage and Noodles

This is another of our family favorites, made countless times. I sometimes add finely chopped chicken to turn it into a one-dish meal.

Serves: 6-8
Overall time 45 minutes

Ingredients:
- 1 (8-ounce) package wheat noodles
- 2 tablespoons butter or olive oil
- 1 cup onion, finely chopped
- 2 cloves garlic, finely chopped

- 4 cups green cabbage, chopped or shredded
- 1½ teaspoons seasoned salt
- ¼ teaspoon black pepper
- ¼-½ cup chicken broth

Directions:
1. Cook noodles according to package directions; drain.
2. Meanwhile, in a large skillet on medium heat, add oil, garlic and onion then cook until softened, about 5 minutes.
3. Add cabbage, seasoned salt, pepper and ¼ cup broth; stir occasionally, adding more broth if needed to retain moisture.
4. Cover; cook over low heat until cabbage is tender, about 30 minutes.
5. Add cooked noodles to cabbage mixture; mix well, stirring until heated throughout.

Macros per Serving & Nutrition Facts
- Calories 394
- Total Fat 10g
- Total Carbohydrate 12g
- Protein 7.3g

Carrot Soufflé V

A light and smooth dish, this makes a great side dish for either formal or informal meals.

Serves: 6
Overall time 50 minutes

Ingredients:
- Carrots (2 cups, peeled, sliced)
- 3 tablespoons whole flour
- ¼ cup softened butter
- 1 teaspoon baking powder
- Eggs (3)
- ½ teaspoon vanilla
- Milk (1 cup)
- ½ teaspoon cinnamon
- Stevia (⅓ cup)

Directions:
1. In a small saucepan, cook carrots in water until tender; drain.
2. Add your carrots to a blender and pulse until soft; add butter, eggs, milk, sugar, flour, baking powder, vanilla, and cinnamon. Blend until smooth.
3. Pour into a greased 8x8-inch casserole dish; bake at 350 degrees for 40 minutes, or until knife inserted in center comes out clean.

Macros per Serving & Nutrition Facts
- Calories 362.8
- Total Fat 10.4g
- Total Carbohydrate 13g
- Protein 8.2g

Candied Sweet Potatoes V 20

This is a quick stovetop version of the traditional baked candied sweet potatoes.

Serves: 6
Overall time 20 minutes

Ingredients:
- 6 medium sweet potatoes, cooked whole and peeled
- 2 tablespoons butter
- ⅔ cup stevia
- ½ cup water
- salt to taste

Directions:
1. Cut cooked, peeled potatoes in half lengthwise; set aside.
2. In a large skillet, melt butter over medium heat; add sugar and stir until sugar is melted.
3. Add water; stir and bring to a boil.

4. Place the sweet potatoes in the skillet, flat-side down, on top of the syrup; cook slowly over low heat, turning so both sides are coated with syrup and warmed throughout.

Macros per Serving & Nutrition Facts
- Calories 275
- Total Fat 8g
- Total Carbohydrate 52g
- Protein 1g

Desserts Recipes

Blueberry Muffins V

Blueberry muffins are an all-time favorite. Either fresh or frozen blueberries work beautifully, and feel free to add extra blueberries to make these muffins bursting with goodness.

Serves: 12
Overall time 25 minutes

Ingredients:
- 1¾ cups whole flour
- ⅓ cup stevia
- 2½ teaspoons baking powder
- ½ teaspoon salt
- ¾ cup milk
- 1 egg, lightly beaten
- ⅓ cup butter, softened
- 1 cup blueberries, fresh or frozen

Directions
1. Heat oven to 400 degrees
2. In a medium bowl, combine salt, baking powder, stevia and flour then set aside.
3. In a large bowl, beat butter and stevia until creamy; add egg and milk.
4. Add flour mixture to butter mixture and stir until the dry ingredients are moistened and a few lumps remain; fold in blueberries.
5. Spoon batter into twelve greased muffin cups; bake at 400 degrees for 18 minutes, or until a toothpick can be inserted in the center and come out clean.

Macros per Serving & Nutrition Facts
- Calories 162.8
- Total Fat 3.4g
- Total Carbohydrate 11.2g
- Protein 7.5g

Tender Stevia Cookies V 20

The buttermilk in this stevia cookie recipe adds moisture and tenderness. These cookies are incredibly soft and very easy for you to digest after chewing thoroughly.

Serves: 24
Overall time 20 minutes

Ingredients:
- 2 cups whole wheat or light baking flour
- ¼ teaspoon salt
- ¾ teaspoon baking soda
- 1 teaspoon cinnamon
- ¼ cup butter, softened
- 1 cup stevia
- 1 egg, lightly beaten
- ½ cup buttermilk
- frosting

Directions:
1. Heat oven to 350 degrees.
2. In a medium bowl, combine flour, salt, baking soda and cinnamon; set aside.
3. In a large bowl, beat butter and stevia together until fluffy; add egg and milk; continue beating until smooth.
4. Stir flour mixture into egg mixture, stirring just until well blended.
5. Drop by tablespoonfuls onto a greased baking sheet, about 2-inches apart.
6. Bake in a 350-degree oven for 10 minutes, or until lightly browned.
7. Lightly spread cooled cookies with frosting.

Macros per Serving & Nutrition Facts
- Calories 73

- Total Fat 5g
- Total Carbohydrate 5g
- Protein 1g

Tomato Juice Cake V

The result is a very moist cake, and no – it does not taste like tomatoes! It won't rise as high as most cakes, so just cut it into bars to serve and eat it like a Texas Sheet Cake or bar cookie.

Serves: 12-15
Overall time 30 minutes

Ingredients:
- 1¼ cups whole wheat or light baking flour
- ½ teaspoon baking soda
- 2 teaspoons baking powder
- ½ teaspoon salt
- 1 teaspoon cinnamon
- ¼ teaspoon cloves
- ¼ teaspoon nutmeg
- ½ teaspoon allspice
- ⅓ cup butter, softened
- ¼ cup applesauce
- ¾ cup stevia
- 2 large eggs
- 1 cup tomato juice
- ½ cup golden raisins (optional)
- ½ cups walnuts, finely ground (optional)
- cream cheese frosting

Direction:
1. Heat oven to 350 degrees and lightly grease a baking dish.
2. In a medium bowl, combine spices, salt, baking powder, flour and baking soda; set aside.

3. In another bowl, beat stevia, applesauce and butter until fluffy. Add eggs individually and continue to beat until incorporated.
4. Add flour mixture alternately with tomato juice and beat until blended; fold in raisins and ground walnuts if desired.
5. Pour batter into your baking dish and set to bake for about 25 minutes, or until a toothpick can be inserted in the cake's center and come out clean. Cool; frost.

Macros per Serving & Nutrition Facts
- Calories 157.5
- Total Fat 3.4g
- Total Carbohydrate 30.9g
- Protein 1.8g

Cheesy Chive Muffins V 20

This is a savory muffin, rather than the common sweet muffin. I make these tasty morsels to eat with light, blended soups, such as tomato or zucchini-potato soup. Need that sweet taste? Try a little honey butter on them.

Serves: 12
Overall time 20 minutes

Ingredients:
- 2 cups whole flour
- 1 teaspoon salt
- 3 teaspoons baking powder
- ½ teaspoon paprika
- 2 eggs, lightly beaten
- 1 cup buttermilk
- ¾ cup milk
- ½ cup cheddar cheese, shredded
- ½ cup Parmesan cheese, grated

- ½ cup vegetable oil
- tablespoons chives, finely chopped

Directions:
1. Heat oven to 350 degrees and lightly grease your muffin tin.
2. In a large bowl, mix flour, salt, baking powder and paprika; set aside.
3. In a medium bowl, add eggs, buttermilk, milk, cheddar cheese, Parmesan cheese and oil; mix well.
4. Pour egg mixture into flour mixture, stirring just until the dry ingredients are moistened and a few lumps remain; stir in chives.
5. Spoon into muffin tin then set to bake for about 15 minutes, or until a toothpick can be inserted in the center and come out clean.

Macros per Serving & Nutrition Facts
- Calories 176.7
- Total Fat 8g
- Total Carbohydrate 19.4g
- Protein 6.6g

Walnut Cake V

Surprisingly light and tender. You don't have to give up the flavor of nuts just because you need soft food.

Serves: 12 - 15
Overall time 40 minutes

Ingredients:
- 3½ cups whole wheat flour
- ¼ teaspoon baking powder
- 2 teaspoons baking soda
- ½ cup stevia
- 4 large eggs

- 1½ cups buttermilk
- ½ cup butter, softened
- 1 teaspoon vanilla
- ½ teaspoon salt
- 1½ cups walnuts, finely ground
- ½ cup vegetable oil
- frosting

Directions:
1. Heat oven to 350 degrees and lightly grease a baking dish.
2. In a bowl, combine salt, baking powder, flour and baking soda; set aside.
3. In another bowl, beat butter, oil and stevia together until smooth; beat in eggs individually, then vanilla.
4. Add flour mixture to egg mixture alternately with buttermilk, beating just until smooth and blended fold in ground walnuts.
5. Pour batter into your baking dish and set to bake for about 35 minutes, or until toothpick can be inserted in the center and come out clean. Cool; frost.

Macros per Serving & Nutrition Facts
- Calories 180
- Total Fat 7g
- Total Carbohydrate 28g
- Protein 2g

Yogurt Spice Bundt Cake V

Delicious. The yogurt makes it moist, the spice gives it just the right flavor. Be sure to use your electric mixer – it helps this cake turn out so light!

Serves: 12-15
Overall time 50 minutes

Ingredients:
- 2 cups whole flour
- 1 teaspoon cinnamon
- 1 teaspoon allspice
- ½ teaspoon nutmeg
- ½ teaspoon salt
- 1½ teaspoons baking soda
- 1¼ cups stevia
- 1 cup butter, softened
- 3 eggs
- 1 cup plain or vanilla yogurt
- 1 teaspoon vanilla
- powdered stevia or frosting

Directions:
1. Heat oven to 325 degrees and lightly grease a bundt pan.
2. In a bowl, combine baking soda, salt, nutmeg, allspice, cinnamon and flour.
3. In another bowl, beat stevia and butter together.
4. Add eggs individually; add yogurt, vanilla, and flour mixture, beating just until blended
5. Pour batter into your prepared pan; set to bake for 45 minutes, or until a toothpick can be inserted in the center of the cake and come out clean.
6. Cool; turn pan upside down over a cake plate to remove cake. Dust top with powdered stevia or frost.

Macros per Serving & Nutrition Facts
- Calories 350
- Total Fat 13g
- Total Carbohydrate 56g
- Protein 4g

Buttermilk Prune Muffins V

You can buy prunes that are already chopped into small bits, or you can use whole pitted prunes and cut them into small pieces. These tasty muffins are wonderful while still warm out of the oven. Try them with honey butter. Delicious.

Serves: 12

Overall time 30 minutes

Ingredients:
- 2 cups water
- 1 cup prune bits
- 5 tablespoons butter, softened
- 3 tablespoons stevia
- 2 eggs, lightly beaten
- 1 cup buttermilk, room temperature
- ½ teaspoon salt
- ½ teaspoon lemon peel powder
- ½ teaspoon cinnamon
- ¾ cup whole wheat flour
- 1¼ cup whole flour
- 1 tablespoon baking powder
- ½ teaspoon baking soda

Directions:
1. Heat oven to 400 degrees
2. In a small saucepan, boil water; remove from heat. Add prunes and let soak for 8 minutes. Drain prunes; sift some of the flour over the prune bits; toss to coat, then set aside.
3. In a large bowl, cream butter and stevia; add eggs and buttermilk.
4. Add salt, lemon powder, cinnamon, flours, baking powder and baking soda, mixing just until the dry ingredients are moistened and a few lumps remain; fold in prunes.
5. Spoon batter into greased muffin cups; bake at 400 degrees for 18 minutes, or until toothpick inserted in center comes out clean.

Macros per Serving & Nutrition Facts

- Calories 194.9
- Total Fat 1.3g
- Total Carbohydrate 121.2g
- Protein 3.8g

Bohemian Apple Kolaches V

I grew up with these delicious fruits filled rolls, made by hand by my grandmother, who grew up in a Bohemian community in Iowa.

Serves: 6
Overall time 1 hr. 40 minutes

Ingredients:
- 2 packages active dry yeast
- ½ cup plus 1 tablespoon stevia
- ¼ cup lukewarm water
- 1¼ cups butter, divided, melted
- 2 cups milk
- 2 whole eggs plus 4 yolks
- 1 ½ teaspoons salt
- ½ teaspoon powdered lemon peel
- 1 teaspoon vanilla
- 6 – 7 cups whole wheat flour

Apple Filling
- 2 cups applesauce
- 1 egg, beaten, reserved
- cinnamon and stevia mixed

Directions:
1. Heat oven to 400 degrees.
2. Dissolve yeast in ¼ cup lukewarm water; add 1 tablespoon stevia, stir. Rest yeast mixture for 5 minutes or until bubbly.
3. Meanwhile, combine 1 cup melted butter and milk in the microwave or a saucepan until warmed (not scalding).

4. In a large bowl, add whole eggs and yolks plus remaining stevia and beat until thickened.
5. Add milk and butter mixture to egg mixture; beat in salt, lemon peel and vanilla.
6. Beat in flour, one cup at a time, until it becomes too thick to beat.
7. Place dough on floured pastry board and knead until smooth, about 5 minutes. Place in greased bowl, rounding up with greased side up. Cover with towel and let rise in a warm place until doubled.
8. Punch down dough; place on a lightly floured board and divide into 6 large pieces. Next cut each of the large pieces into 12 smaller pieces; form each into balls.
9. Place balls on a baking sheet and brush each with melted butter; cover and let rise again until double.
10. Press the center of each down, making a flat indentation in the center, and fill each with 1 tablespoon applesauce; let rise again, about 30 minutes.
11. Bake in a 400-degree oven for 7 to 10 minutes or just until lightly browned; sprinkle with cinnamon stevia.

Macros per Serving & Nutrition Facts
- Calories 60.6
- Total Fat 4.2g
- Total Carbohydrate 5g
- Protein 0.7g

Banana Pineapple Bread V

The pineapple gives this bread a very nice flavor. While pineapple is a rather chewy fruit, the crushed pineapple baked into this bread makes for an easy chew. However, if even crushed pineapple is difficult for you, just try one of the other delicious breads.

Serves: 8

Overall time 1 hour 10 minutes

Ingredients:
- 1 cups coconut flour
- Baking soda, 1 tsp.
- 2 teaspoons baking powder
- ½ teaspoon salt
- ⅓ cup butter, softened
- ¼ cup applesauce
- ¼ cup granulated stevia
- ¼ cup brown stevia
- 2 eggs
- 1 cup banana, mashed
- Pineapple, canned, 8oz, crushed, undrained

Directions:
1. Heat oven to 350 degrees
2. In a bowl, combine salt, baking powder and flour; set aside.
3. Cream together butter, applesauce, and stevia; add eggs and mix well.
4. Add flour mixture to egg mixture, stirring just until the dry ingredients are moistened and a few lumps remain; fold in mashed banana and pineapple in juice.
5. Pour into a greased 9x5-inch loaf pan.
6. Bake in prepared oven for about 60 minutes, or until done.

Macros per Serving & Nutrition Facts
- Calories 214.2
- Total Fat 6.4g
- Total Carbohydrate 13g
- Protein 5.3g

Tapioca Pudding V

This has always been my mother's favorite pudding, so it's been made often at our house.
Serves: 6
Overall time 1 hour 30 minutes

Ingredients:
- 4 cups milk
- ⅓ cup tapioca
- 3 eggs
- 1 cup stevia
- 1 teaspoon vanilla
- whipped cream (optional)

Directions:
1. In a medium saucepan, heat milk until near boiling; reduce heat and add tapioca, cook on low heat for 20 minutes, or until tapioca is translucent. Stir occasionally.
2. In a small bowl, beat eggs, stevia and vanilla together; slowly add egg mixture to saucepan; continue cooking over low heat and stirring constantly until pudding thickens to desired consistency.
3. Refrigerate to chill. Top each serving with whipped cream if desired.

Macros per Serving & Nutrition Facts
- Calories 140
- Total Fat 3.1g
- Total Carbohydrate 24g
- Protein 4g

Conclusion

There you have it! Together we have explored 74 amazingly simple recipes that you can enjoy within Stage 3 of recovery from a bariatric surgery. We are elated that you were able to stick with us to the end and hope you will consider joining us again when we explore Stage 4 of the bariatric surgery recovery diet.

Achieving a speedy and successful recovery is vital right now, and we want to continue to help you get there. So, be sure to stick to all the guidelines presented in this book and be sure to leave us a positive review if you enjoyed what you read. Until next time, good luck, and have a speedy recovery.

Bariatric Cookbook
Stage 4

80 Delicious Breakfast, Lunch, Dinner, Snack and Desert
Recipes You Can Enjoy in Stage 4 Post Weight Loss Surgery

Table of Contents

Introduction

Congratulations, once again, on successfully completing your gastric sleeve surgery and making it successfully into your final stage of the recovery diet! Up to this point you have conquered eating on a standard meal plan that consists of soft solids. Now, we will be entering into the final phase of your diet, you guessed it! This is the 'Regular Foods' stage of your recovery diet.

Before you proceed to this stage it is important that you check your consumption log and ask yourself if you can comfortably consume a minimum of 12ozs of food daily without experiencing added pouch irritation, discomfort, and vomiting? If so, then great; feel free to move on to stage 4 confidently. However, if you are still not quite there, don't rush yourself. Instead, consider sticking to stage 3 for a few more days to a week until you are able to comfortably move on. Remember, every patient is different so your body may heal differently than others. Listen to your body and adjust your recovery process to suit your body and specific needs.

So, what should you expect to achieve in Stage 4?

In this stage of your diet you will be introducing regular foods to your diet. This will include high fiber foods, fruits, vegetables as well as foods rich in protein such as low fat dairy products, beans, egg and lean meat. In terms of carbs you are allowed to moderately enjoy a small serving of whole grains. By keeping your carb intake to a minimum and indulging in more protein-filled, high fiber foods you will be able to stay fuller for longer hence aiding in not only your recovery but also your weight loss journey. With this in mind you are free to explore different foods just as long you keep your meals low in both fat and sugar while watching your portions.

General Guidelines of Stage 4:

- Try to slowly introduce yourself to foods of all the major food groups to achieve somewhat of a balanced diet.
- Try to drink a glass of liquid about 30 minutes before having a meal so that you won't need to drink anything in the minutes leading up to the meal then waiting at least another 30 minutes after eating to have a drink.
- Your goal for each day will be to aim for a standard meal plan of 3 meals with 2 snacks daily. Feel free to use protein shakes as your snacks or even as meal replacements from time to time.
- Pace yourself while eating and ensure that you chew your food thoroughly.
- Try to stick to only healthy foods as much as possible, starting with protein (eating at least 60g of protein daily).

- Start out with small portion sizes and gradually move up as you see fit. Listen to your body! Every patient is different so, don't beat yourself up if you find that you can't tolerate eating 6oz of food all at once. Just pace yourself and start with a smaller portion at a time.
- Remember to take your vitamins

- Continue to drink at least 64oz of low-calorie fluids daily

- Avoid sugary and caffeinated drinks like soda or coffee

- Remember all the guidelines and tips that you have come to practice from the 3 previous stages.

This is a lot of information to take in, but it really isn't as complicated as it sounds. Try to just take it a step at a time and be mindful of what your body is telling you as you go. Be sure to consult your doctor should you experience long periods of vomiting or any adverse reactions for an extended period of time. Of course, try to stick to the guidelines as best as possible so that you can avoid any adverse reactions and continue on a healthy path to recovery.

In this Bariatric Cookbook, we are going to help keep you on track with 80 Delicious recipe suggestions that you can enjoy in Stage 4 of your post gastric sleeve recovery diet. We guarantee that once you see how simple it can be things will begin to become clearer. So, without further ado, let's get started.

Breakfast Recipes

Veggie Quiche Muffins V

These quiche muffins will knock your boots off. They are filled with protein and will keep you filled until your next planned meal.

Serves: 12
Overall time: 50 minutes

Ingredients:
- Cheddar (3/4 cup, low-fat, shredded)
- Green Onion (1 cup, chopped)
- Broccoli (1 cup, chopped)
- Tomatoes (1 cup, diced)
- Milk (2 cups, non-fat)
- Eggs (4)
- Pancake mix (1 cup)
- Oregano (1 tsp.)
- Salt (1/2 tsp.)
- Pepper (1/2 tsp.)

Directions:
1. Set your oven to preheat to 375 degrees F, and lightly grease a 12-cup muffin tin with oil.
2. Sprinkle your tomatoes, broccoli, onions, and cheddar into your muffin cups.
3. Combine your remaining ingredients in a medium, whisk to combine then pour evenly on top of your veggies.
4. Set to bake in your preheated oven for about 40 minutes or until golden brown.
5. Allow to cool slightly (about 5 minutes) then serve. Enjoy!

Macros per Serving & Nutrition Facts
- Calories 58.8
- Total Fat 3.2 g
- Total Carbohydrate 2.9 g
- Protein 5.1g

Steel Cut Oat Blueberry Pancakes V 20

These delicious oat blueberry pancakes are simply delicious with berries! They are soft and very easy on the stomach.

Serves: 4
Overall time: 20 minutes

Ingredients:
- Water (1 ½ cups)
- Oats (½ cup, steel cut)
- Salt (1/8 tsp.)
- Flour (1 cup, whole wheat)
- Baking powder (½ tsp.)
- Baking soda (½ tsp.)
- Egg (1)
- Milk (1 cup)
- Greek yogurt (½ cup, vanilla)
- Blueberries (1 cup, frozen)
- Agave Nectar (½ cup + 2 tbsp.)

Directions:
1. Combine your oats, salt, and water together in a medium saucepan, stir, and allow to come to a boil over high heat.
2. Lower heat, and allow to simmer for about 10 min, or until oats get tender. Set aside.
3. Combine all your remaining ingredients, except agave nectar, in a medium bowl then fold in oats.
4. Preheat your griddle, and lightly grease. Cook ¼ cup of batter at a time for about 3 minutes per side.
5. Garnish with agave.

Macros per Serving & Nutrition Facts
- Calories 257
- Total Fat 7 g
- Total Carbohydrate 46 g
- Protein 14 g

Very Berry Muesli V

This Very Berry Muesli is a delicious soft cereal based breakfast dish that is healthy, delicious and perfect for this stage.

Serves: 2
Overall time: 6 hours

Ingredients:
- Oats (1 cup, old-fashioned, rolled)
- Yogurt (1 cup, fruit flavored)
- Milk (1/2 cup, 1%)
- Salt (1/8 tsp.)
- Raisins (1/2 cup, dried)
- Apple (1/2 cup, chopped, cored)
- Blueberries (1/2 cup, frozen)
- Walnuts (1/4 cup, chopped, toasted)

Directions:
1. Combine your yogurt, salt, and oats together in a medium bowl, mix well, then cover the mixture tightly.
2. Allow to rest in the refrigerator for at least 6 hours.
3. Add your raisins, and apples the gently fold.
4. Top with walnuts and serve. Enjoy!

Macros per Serving & Nutrition Facts
- Calories 195
- Total Fat 4 g
- Total Carbohydrate 31 g
- Protein 6 g

Strawberry & Mushroom Breakfast Sandwich V 20

Having fruits for breakfast is a brilliant way to get in your fruit count for the day in a simple yet delicious way.

Serves: 4
Overall time: 10 minutes

Ingredients:
- Cream cheese (8 oz., low fat, softened)
- Honey (1 tbsp.)
- Lemon zest (1 tbsp., grated)
- Portobello Mushrooms (4, sliced, toasted)
- Strawberries (2 cups, sliced)

Directions:
1. Add your honey, lemon zest, and cheese to a food processor, and process until fully incorporated.
2. Use your cheese mixture to spread on your mushrooms as you would butter.
3. Top with strawberries. Enjoy!

Macros per Serving & Nutrition Facts
- Calories 180
- Total Fat 16 g
- Total Carbohydrate 6 g
- Protein 2 g

Turkey Sausage and Mushroom Strata

If you have never had a Mushroom Strata before then this recipe is about to change your life. Its filling, easy to digest and great for your weight loss journey.

Serves: 12
Overall time: 1 hour 15 minutes

Ingredients:

- Ciabatta bread (8 oz., wheat, cubed)
- Turkey sausage (12 oz., chopped)
- Milk (2 cups, fat free)
- Cheddar (4 oz., low-fat, shredded)
- Eggs (3 large)
- Egg substitute (12 oz.)
- Green onion (½ cup, chopped)
- Mushroom (1 cup, sliced)
- Paprika (½ tsp.)
- Pepper (1/2 tsp.)
- Parmesan cheese (2 tbsp., grated)

Directions:
1. Set oven to preheat to 400 degrees F. Lay your bread cubes flat on a baking tray and set it to toast for about 8 min.
2. Meanwhile, add a skillet over medium heat with sausage, and allow to cook, while stirring, until fully brown and crumbled.
3. In a large bowl add salt, pepper, paprika, parmesan cheese, egg substitute, eggs, cheddar cheese, and milk, then whisk to combine.
4. Add in your remaining ingredients and toss well to incorporate. Transfer mixture to a large baking dish (preferably a 9x13-inch) then tightly cover and allow to rest in the refrigerator overnight.
5. Set your oven to preheat to 350 degrees, remove the cover from your casserole and set to bake until fully cooked and golden brown.
6. Slice and serve.

Macros per Serving & Nutrition Facts
- Calories 180
- Total Fat 16 g
- Total Carbohydrate 9 g
- Protein 2 g

Sweet Millet Congee V

A congee is much like a filling porridge, this Sweet Millet Congee leaves you feeling satisfied and filled with enough energy to carry on with your day.

Serves: 4
Overall time: 2 hours 15 minutes

Ingredients:
- Millet (1 cup, hulled, rinsed, drained)
- Water (5 cups)
- Sweet potato (1 cup, peeled, diced)
- Cinnamon (1 tsp., ground)
- Stevia (2 tbsp.)
- Apple (1 medium, diced)
- Honey (¼ cup)

Directions:
1. In a deep pot, add your stevia, sweet potato, cinnamon, water, and millet then stir to combine.
2. Allow to come to a boil over high heat then reduce to a simmer on low.
3. Cook like this for about an hour, on until your water is fully absorbed and millet is cooked.
4. Stir in your remaining ingredients and serve.

Macros per Serving & Nutrition Facts
- Calories 136
- Total Fat 1 g
- Total Carbohydrate 28.5 g
- Protein 3.1 g

Summer Breakfast Quinoa Bowls V

These Quinoa bowls are tasty, filling and packed with protein.

Serves: 2
Overall time: 28 minutes

Ingredients:
- Peach (1 small, sliced)
- Quinoa (1/3 cup, rinsed)
- Low fat milk (2/3 + 3/4 cup)
- Vanilla extract (1/2 tsp.)
- Natural stevia (2 tsp.)
- Raspberries (12, fresh)
- Blueberries (14, fresh)
- Honey (2 tsp.)

Directions:
1. Add natural stevia, 2/3 cup milk, and quinoa to a saucepan, and stir to combine.
2. Bring to a boil over medium heat then cover and reduce heat to a low simmer.
3. Continue to cook for about 20 minutes (you should be able to fluff quinoa with a fork).
4. Grease and preheat your grill to medium and grill your peach slices for about a minute per side then set aside.
5. Reheat your remaining milk in the microwave and set aside.
6. Split your cooked quinoa evenly between 2 serving bowls and top evenly with your remaining ingredients. Enjoy!

Macros per Serving & Nutrition Facts
- Calories 180
- Total Fat 4 g
- Total Carbohydrate 36 g
- Protein 4.5 g

Perfect Granola V

Granola makes the perfect grab and go breakfast. It's light yet nutritional and very tasty.

Serves: 10
Overall time: 40 minutes

Ingredients:
- Canola oil (1/4 cup)
- Honey (4 tbsp.)
- Vanilla (1 ½ tsp.)
- Old fashioned rolled oats (6 cups)
- Almond (1 cup, slivered)
- Unsweetened coconut (1/2 cup shredded)
- Bran flakes (2 cups)
- Walnuts (3/4 cup, chopped)
- Raisins (1 cup)
- Cooking spray (parchment paper can also be used)

Directions:
1. Prepare oven to preheat at 325 degrees F.
2. In a saucepan cook oil and vanilla gently over low flame, occasionally stirring for roughly 5 mins.
3. Place all (except raisins) ingredients remaining, in a large bowl and combine.
4. Stir in honey and oil mixture slowly and ensure that all grains are properly coated.
5. Cover a baking tray with parchment paper or use cooking spray to spray it lightly.
6. Spread cereal evenly in the tray and bake for 25 mins. (occasionally stirring to keep mixture from burning), or until very lightly browned, or the grains crisp.
7. When finished, remove cereal and put to cool.
8. Add the cup of raisins and mix well so that raisins are thoroughly spread through the grain mixture.

Macros per Serving & Nutrition Facts
- Calories 458
- Total Fat 21 g
- Total Carbohydrate 62 g
- Protein 12.1 g

Spinach, Mushroom, and Feta Cheese Scramble V 20

This delicious scramble combines creamy scrambled eggs with delicious wilted spinach and filing mushrooms.

Serves: 1
Overall time: 10 minutes

Ingredients:
- Olive oil cooking spray
- Mushroom (½ cup, fresh, sliced)
- Spinach (1 cup, fresh, chopped)
- Eggs (1 whole)
- Egg whites (2 eggs)
- Feta cheese (2 tbsp.)
- Pepper (to taste)

Directions:
1. Set a lightly greased, medium skillet over medium heat. Add spinach, and mushrooms, and cook until spinach wilts.
2. Combine egg whites, cheese, pepper, and whole egg together in a medium bowl then whisk to combine.
3. Pour into your skillet and cook, while stirring, until set (about 4 minutes). Serve.

Macros per Serving & Nutrition Facts
- Calories 236.5
- Total Fat 11.4 g
- Total Carbohydrate 12.9 g

- Protein 22.2 g

Refrigerator Overnight Oatmeal V

Overnight oatmeal will become your new favorite breakfast dish. It's easy to make, creamy, thick and filling.

Serves: 2
Overall time: 9 minutes

Ingredients:
- Oats (1 cup, old fashioned)
- Non-fat yogurt (1 cup, vanilla)
- Milk (½ cup, non-fat)
- Blueberries (1 cup, frozen)
- Chia seeds (1 tbsp.)

Directions:
1. Add all your ingredients to a medium mixing bowl, and stir.
2. Split evenly among 2 airtight containers, seal, and refrigerate overnight. Serve.

Macros per Serving & Nutrition Facts
- Calories 244
- Total Fat 5 g
- Total Carbohydrate 37 g
- Protein 16 g

Red Velvet Pancakes with Cream Cheese Topping V 20

Just because food is healthy doesn't mean it has to be dull. This fun and delicious recipe for red velvet pancakes will blow your mind.

Serves: 2
Overall time: 30 minutes

Ingredients:
Cream Cheese Topping:
- Cream cheese (2 oz.)
- Yogurt (3 tbsp., plain, fat free)
- Honey (3 tbsp.)
- Milk (1 tbsp., fat-free)

Pancakes:
- Flour (½ cup, whole wheat flour)
- Flour (½ cup, all-purpose)
- Baking powder (2 ¼ tsp.)
- Cocoa powder (½ tbsp., unsweetened)
- Salt (¼ tsp.)
- Stevia (1/8 cup)
- Egg (1 large)
- Milk (1 cup + 2 tbsp., fat-free)
- Vanilla (1 tsp.)
- Red paste food coloring (1 tsp.)

Directions:
1. Combine all your topping ingredients in a medium bowl and set aside.
2. Add all your pancake ingredients together in a large bowl and fold until combined.
3. Set a greased skillet over medium heat to get hot. Add ¼ cup of pancake batter onto the hot skillet and cook until bubbles begin to form on the top.
4. Flip and cook until set. Repeat until your batter is done. Add your toppings and serve.

Macros per Serving & Nutrition Facts
- Calories 231
- Total Fat 4 g
- Total Carbohydrate 43 g
- Protein 7 g

Lunch Recipes

Fresh Shrimp Spring Rolls V 20

These springs rolls are more like summer rolls. They are gluten free, delicious and goes great with a refreshing glass of sugar free lemonade.

Serves: 12
Overall time: 20 minutes

Ingredients:
- Rice paper (12 sheets)
- Bib lettuce (12 leaves, washed)
- Basil (12 leaves, washed)
- Cilantro (¾ cup, fresh, washed)
- Carrots (1 cup, shredded, washed)
- Cucumber (½ medium, thinly sliced)
- Shrimp (20oz., cooked, de-veined and peeled)

Directions:
1. Add all your vegetables, and shrimp to separate bowls and lay out on a flat surface.
2. Set a damp paper towel tower flat on your work surface.
3. Quickly wet one of your rice papers under warm water and lay on paper towel.
4. Top with 1 of each vegetable, and 4 pieces of shrimp, then roll your rice paper into a burrito – like roll.
5. Repeat until all your vegetables and shrimp has been used up. Serve, and enjoy.

Macros per Serving & Nutrition Facts
- Calories 67
- Total Fat 2.9 g
- Total Carbohydrate 7.4 g
- Protein 2.6 g

Sunshine Wrap

This citrusy wrap is filled with the perfect mixture of savory and sweet to keep you enticed and looking forward to lunch.

Serves: 2
Overall time: 30 minutes

Ingredients:
- Grilled chicken breast (8oz., cubed)
- Celery (½ cup, diced)
- Mandarin oranges (2/3 cup, wedges)
- Onion (¼ cup, minced)
- Mayonnaise (2 tbsp.)
- Soy sauce (1 tsp.)
- Garlic powder (¼ tsp.)
- Black pepper (¼ tsp.)
- Tortilla (1 large, whole wheat)
- Lettuce leaves (4 large, cleaned)

Directions:
1. Combine all your ingredients, except tortilla, and lettuce in a large bowl and toss to evenly coat.
2. Lay your tortillas down on a flat surface and cut into quarters.
3. Top each quarter with a lettuce leaf and spoon your chicken mixture into the middle of each.
4. Roll each tortilla into a cone and seal by slightly wetting the edge with water. Enjoy!

Macros per Serving & Nutrition Facts
- Calories 280.8
- Total Fat 21.1 g
- Total Carbohydrate 3 g
- Protein 19 g

Sweet Roasted Beet & Arugula Tortilla Pizza V

If you love pizza, then why not have the best of both worlds. Enjoy a healthy slice of deliciousness with this easy to follow recipe.

Serves: 6
Overall time: 25 minutes

Ingredients:
- Beets (2 small, roasted, chopped)
- Corn Tortillas (6)
- Arugula (1 cup)
- Goat cheese (½ cup)
- Blackberries (1 cup)
- Honey (2 tbsp.)
- Balsamic vinegar (2 tbsp.)

Directions:
1. Set your oven to preheat to 350 F. Lay your tortillas on a flat surface.
2. Top with beets, berries, and goat cheese. Combine your balsamic vinegar, and honey together in a small bowl, and whisk to combine.
3. Drizzle the mixture over your pizza, and to bake for about 10 minutes, or until your cheese has melted slightly, and your tortilla crisp.
4. Garnish with arugula and serve.

Macros per Serving & Nutrition Facts
- Calories 286
- Total Fat 40 g
- Total Carbohydrate 42 g
- Protein 15 g

Southwestern Black Bean Cakes with Guacamole V

It is said that bacon makes everything better but, in this recipe, dear I say it, it's the Guac that makes it really worthwhile.

Serves: 4
Overall time: 25 minutes

Ingredients:
- Whole wheat bread crumbs (1 cup)
- Cilantro (3 tbsp., fresh, chopped)
- Garlic (2 cloves)
- Black beans (15 oz. can, low sodium)
- Chipotle peppers in Adobo sauce (7 oz. can)
- Cumin (1 tsp., ground)
- Egg (1 large)
- Avocado (½ medium, diced)
- Lime juice (1 tbsp.)
- Tomato (1 small, plum)

Directions:
1. Drain beans then add all your ingredients, except avocado, lime juice, and eggs, to a food processor and run until the mixture begin to pull away from the sides of processor.
2. Transfer to a large bowl and add in egg then mix well.
3. Form into 4 even patties, and cook on a preheated, greased grill over medium heat for about 10 minutes, flipping halfway through.
4. Add your avocado, and lime juice in a small bowl, then stir and mash together using a fork.
5. Season to taste then serve with bean cakes.

Macros per Serving & Nutrition Facts
- Calories 178
- Total Fat 7 g
- Total Carbohydrate 25 g
- Protein 11 g

Veggie Quesadillas with Cilantro Yogurt Dip V

Quesadillas make great snacks but if portioned well they can also serve as a delicious lunch dish.

Serves: 3
Overall time: 25 minutes

Ingredients:
- Black Beans (1 cup)
- Cilantro (2 tbsp., chopped)
- Bell pepper (½, finely chopped)
- Corn kernels (½ cup)
- Cheese (1 cup, low-fat, shredded)
- Corn tortillas (6, soft)
- Carrot (1 medium, shredded)

Directions:
1. Set your skillet to preheat on low heat. Lay 3 tortillas on a flat surface.
2. Top evenly with peppers, carrots, cilantro, beans, corn, and cheese over the tortillas (covering each with another tortilla, maximum.
3. Add your quesadilla to your preheated skillet, and cook until the cheese melts, and tortilla becomes a nice golden brown (about 2 min).
4. Flip to quesadilla and cook for about a minute (or until golden).
5. Mix well. Slice each quesadilla into 4 even wedges and serve with your dip. Enjoy!

Macros per Serving & Nutrition Facts
- Calories 344
- Total Fat 8 g
- Total Carbohydrate 46 g
- Protein 27 g

Mayo-less Tuna Salad 20

This tuna salad is low in fat but still carries the punch you expect of a tuna salad.

Serves: 2
Overall time: 5 minutes

Ingredients:
- Tuna (5 oz., light, in water, drained)
- Olive oil (1 tbsp., extra virgin)
- Red wine vinegar (1 tbsp.)
- Green onion (¼ cup, chopped)
- Arugula (2 cups)
- Pasta (1 cup, cooked)
- Parmesan cheese (1 tbsp., shaved)
- Black pepper

Directions:
1. Combine all your ingredients into a medium bowl. Split mixture between two plates. Serve, and enjoy.

Macros per Serving & Nutrition Facts
- Calories 213.2
- Total Fat 6.2 g
- Total Carbohydrate 20.3 g
- Protein 22.7 g

Southwest Style Zucchini Rice Bowl 20

This zucchini rice bowl topped with salsa, sour cream and cheese that goes brilliantly with the chicken breast and vegetables that makes it the perfect meal.

Serves: 2

Overall time: 12 minutes
Ingredients:
- Vegetable oil (1 tbsp.)
- Chopped vegetables (1 cup, of your choice)
- Chicken breast (1 cup, grilled, chopped)
- Zucchini rice (1 cup, cooked)
- Salsa (4 tbsp.)
- Cheddar cheese (2 tbsp., shredded)
- Sour cream (2 tbsp., low fat)

Directions:
1. Set a skillet with oil to heat up over medium heat.
2. Add chopped vegetables and allow to cook, while stirring, until vegetables become fork tender.
3. Add chicken, and zucchini rice and continue to cook, while stirring, until fully heated through.
4. Split between 2 serving bowls, and garnish with your remaining ingredients. Serve, and enjoy!

Macros per Serving & Nutrition Facts
- Calories 168
- Total Fat 8.2 g
- Total Carbohydrate 18 g
- Protein 5.5 g

Pesto & Mozzarella Stuffed Portobello Mushroom Caps V

When trying to eat only healthy carbs, mushrooms quickly become a staple in your diet. This recipe allows you to use the actual caps and stuff them with cheese and pesto.

Serves: 2
Overall time: 30 minutes

Ingredients:
- Mushrooms (2, Portobello caps, cleaned, stems removed)
- Tomato (1 small, Roma, diced)
- Pesto (2 tbsp.)
- Mozzarella cheese (¼ cup, shredded, low- fat)

Directions:
1. Spoon your pesto into evenly into your mushroom caps, then to with your remaining ingredients.
2. Set to bake at 400 degrees F for about 15 minutes. Enjoy!

Macros per Serving & Nutrition Facts
- Calories 112
- Total Fat 5.4 g
- Total Carbohydrate 7.5 g
- Protein 10.5 g

Pear, Turkey and Cheese Mushroom Sandwich 20

These sandwiches will definitely brighten your day. It's the perfect ratio of serving portions and nutrients.

Serves: 2
Overall time: 9 minutes

Ingredients:
- Mushroom (2 halved, portobello)
- Mustard (2 tsp., Dijon-style)
- Smoked Turkey (2 slices, reduced-sodium)
- Pear (1, cored, thinly sliced)
- Mozzarella cheese (1/4 cup, shredded, low fat)
- Pepper (1/8 tsp., coarsely ground)

Directions:

1. Use your mustard to spread on both slices of mushrooms, then top each side with turkey and set one side aside.
2. Top your remaining half with pear slices, and season with pepper.
3. Close your sandwich, and set to broil for about 3 minutes, or until your cheese has been melted, and turkey warmed. Enjoy!

Macros per Serving & Nutrition Facts
- Calories 337.3
- Total Fat 11.6 g
- Total Carbohydrate 55.8 g
- Protein 16.5 g

Salmon Salad Pita 20

Though not common whole wheat pitas are delicious and when topped with the salmon salad in this recipe it's just superb.

Serves: 3
Overall time: 5 minutes

Ingredients:
- Salmon (¾ cup, Alaskan)
- Yogurt (3 tbsp., plain, fat free)
- Lemon juice (1 tbsp.)
- Bell pepper (2 tbsp., red, minced)
- Red Onion (1 tbsp., minced)
- Capers (1 tsp., rinsed, chopped)
- Dill (1 tsp, dried)
- Lettuce (3 leaves)
- Black pepper (to taste)
- Pita bread (3 small, whole wheat)

Directions:

1. In a bowl, create your salmon salad by combining your first 8 ingredients, then stir.
2. Create salmon pita by spooning your salmon salad evenly onto your letter leaf then placing it inside your pitas. Enjoy!

Macros per Serving & Nutrition Facts
- Calories 239
- Total Fat 7 g
- Total Carbohydrate 19 g
- Protein 25 g

Thai Tofu Quinoa Bowl

These bowls are both filling and delicious. Best of all they are filled with protein and is easy on the stomach.

Serves: 8
Overall time: 1 hour 40 minutes

Ingredients:
- 2 packages (15 ounces each) extra firm tofu, diced
- 2 tablespoons sesame oil
- 3 cups chicken broth
- 2 cups carrots, shredded
- 1 cup fresh cilantro
- 4 tablespoons soy sauce
- 2 cups uncooked quinoa, rinsed
- 1 cup almonds, slivered
- 1 1/3 cups scallions, chopped

For the sauce:
- 4 teaspoons creamy peanut butter
- 4 tablespoons rice wine vinegar
- 1 tablespoon stevia
- Juice of a lime
- 4 tablespoons Sriracha sauce

- 1/3 cup coconut milk
- 2 cloves garlic, minced
- 2 teaspoons ginger, grated

Directions:

1. Rinse and drain the tofu about 30-40 minutes before cooking.
2. Wrap with a kitchen towel and place on a rimmed plate. Place something heavy on it like a heavy bottomed pan so that excess moisture in it is pressed out.
3. Set aside for 15-20 minutes. Chop into pieces.
4. Place tofu in a bowl. Pour soy sauce and sesame oil on it. Toss well. Transfer the tofu on to a lined baking sheet in a single layer.
5. Bake in a preheated oven at 350 F for 30-40 minutes or until crisp. Toss frequently while it is baking.
6. Place a pan over medium heat. Add quinoa and toast it until it turns golden brown. Add broth and stir.
7. Lower heat and cover with a lid. Simmer until all the broth is absorbed.
8. Uncover and fluff with a fork. Set aside.
9. Make the sauce as follows: Add peanut butter to a microwave safe bowl. Microwave on high for 10-12 seconds until it melts.
10. Remove the bowl from the microwave and add rest of the ingredients of the sauce and whisk well. Set aside.

Macros per Serving & Nutrition Facts

- Calories 298
- Total Fat 22.9 g
- Total Carbohydrate 0.4 g
- Protein 22.4 g

One-Skillet Peanut Chicken

This combination of ingredients will surely work for you add bring new flavors in your life.

Serving Size: 4
Overall Time: 30 min
Ingredients:
- 1-pound chicken breast
- 2 tablespoons soy sauce
- 3 tablespoons water
- 2 cloves garlic, chopped
- 1 tablespoon ginger paste
- 2 tablespoons cooking oil
- ½ cup salsa
- 2 ½ tablespoons butter
- 3 green onions, finely chopped

Directions:
1. Cut chicken breasts horizontally in the shape of cutlets and cut them again in half.
2. In a bowl add garlic, soy sauce, water, ginger paste. Add this sauce to chicken and toss to combine, let to marinade for 30 minutes.
3. Meanwhile, combine salsa, and butter. Set aside.
4. Heat oil in a pan and fry chicken pieces until nicely golden from both sides.
5. Now add in salsa mixture and cook covered on low till chicken is done.
6. Garnish green onions and serve with rice.

Macros per Serving & Nutrition Facts
- Calories 259
- Total Fat 4.9g
- Total Carbohydrate 12.6g
- Protein 42.5g

Turkey Stuffed Zucchini Boats – Italian Style

This uniquely presented recipe is going to blow your mind.

Serving Size: 4
Overall Time: 2hrs
Ingredients:
- 1/4 cup soy sauce
- 1 tbsp. canola oil
- 2 tsp sesame oil
- 1 Tbsp. ginger paste
- 2 garlic cloves, minced
- 2 lb. flat iron or flank steak
- 1/4 cup rice vinegar
- 1/8 cup stevia
- ¼ tsp. red pepper flakes
- 4 cups thinly sliced cabbage
- a few green onions, chopped

Directions:
1. Pre-heat oven to 375F.
2. Discard the inner portion of zucchini.
3. Transfer spaghetti sauce in zucchini boats.
4. Bake for about 15-20 minutes.
5. Add some cheese if you like and bake again for ten minutes.
6. Directions for making the sauce:
7. In a pot add ground turkey and cook for 10-12 minutes.
8. Heat oil in pan and cook onion with green pepper for 4-5 minutes. Now add in garlic. Cook for another1-2 minutes by stirring.
9. Drizzle in wine and cook for about four minutes.
10. Transfer of crushed tomatoes, a jar of marinara, thyme, paste, stevia, bay leaves, oregano, crushed pepper flakes, and some salt, simmer for few minutes.
11. Add in cooked meat. Cook covered for 30 minutes.
12. Enjoy.

Macros per Serving & Nutrition Facts
- Calories 52
- Total Fat 2.9g
- Total Carbohydrate 5.6g
- Protein 1.1g

Tomato Baked Tilapia with Lemon

This delicious fish is best for you evening gathering.

Serving Size: 4
Overall Time: 30 mins

Ingredients:
- 4 tilapia fillets
- 2 tbsp. olive oil
- 1 tbsp. fresh basil, chopped
- 1 tbsp. salt
- 1 large tomato thinly sliced
- 1 tbsp. lemon zest
- Salt & Pepper to taste
- ¼ teaspoon lime juice

Directions:
1. Preheat oven to 400F
2. Brush baking tray with cooking oil.
3. Spread fish fillets in the tray.
4. Sprinkle them with salt and pepper.
5. Now place tomato slices, basil, and garlic on fillets.
6. Drizzle them with olive oil.
7. Sprinkle more salt and pepper and drizzle lemon juice.
8. Bake for about 20 minutes.
9. Cook on Broil for 5-10 minutes.

Macros per Serving & Nutrition Facts
- Calories 236
- Total Fat 5g
- Total Carbohydrate 12g
- Protein 18.3g

Stuffed Poblano Peppers 20

Poblano peppers are not as spicy which makes them the perfect vessel for stuffing. This particular recipe utilizes Mexican ingredients for a filling meal.

Serves: 4
Overall time: 30 minutes

Ingredients:
- Poblano peppers (14, seeded, broiled)
- Zucchini rice (½ cup, cooked)
- Grilled Salsa (1½ cups, fresh)
- Black bean (15 oz., rinsed, drained)
- Corn (1½ cup, frozen)
- Cumin (1 tsp.)
- Chili powder (1 tsp.)
- Cayenne pepper (1/8 tsp.)
- Pepper (to taste)
- Mexican cheese (½ cup, shredded)

Directions:
1. Add all your ingredients, except peppers, and ½ of your cheese to a large microwave safe bowl, stir and place to warm for about 3 minutes, stopping to stir every 30 seconds.
2. Spoon your mixture into your peppers and top with remaining cheese.
3. Set to broil on high until cheese melts (about 3 min). Enjoy!

Macros per Serving & Nutrition Facts
- Calories 260
- Total Fat 6 g
- Total Carbohydrate 4g
- Protein 20.5 g

Whole Wheat BLT

Adding a splash of liquid spoke into the bag before sealing will add a more of a BBQ feel to your BLT.

Serves: 3
Overall time: 4 hrs. 40 mins.

Ingredients:
- 1 package thick-cut Turkey bacon in original vacuum-sealed packaging
- 6 slices whole wheat bread, toasted
- 6 slices tomato
- 3 leaves lettuce
- 3 tablespoons mayonnaise

Directions:
1. Preheat the water bath to 140 degrees F. Place sealed Turkey bacon in the water bath.
2. Cook at least 4 hours or overnight. After at least 4 hours, remove Turkey bacon from pan.
3. Brown in the hot pan on both sides. Drain on paper towel.
4. Spread mayonnaise on bread. Assemble sandwiches with tomato and lettuce. Serve.

Macros per Serving & Nutrition Facts
- Calories 812
- Total Fat 70.07g
- Total Carbohydrate 22.56g
- Protein 22.74g

Massaman Curry Chicken with Sweet Potatoes & Peas

Here is a greet treat for all those who love to enjoy curry chicken.

Serving Size: 4
Overall Time: 1 hr.

Ingredients:
- 6 chicken thighs
- 2 medium onions, diced
- 2 sweet potatoes, cubed
- 1 cup peas
- 2 cups chicken broth
- 1 can coconut milk
- 1 cup water
- juice of 1 lime
- 3 tbsp. Curry Paste
- 1 tbsp. olive oil
- salt and pepper to taste
- 2 tbsp. cilantro, chopped
- 2 tbsp. toasted chopped cashews

Directions:
1. Heat olive oil in a saucepan.
2. Sprinkle drumsticks with salt and some pepper.
3. Cook in oil until nicely browned. Remove.
4. Add the curry paste. Let to cook until smoked.
5. Now transfer onions and cook for 5 minutes.
6. Add chicken again to the pan.
7. Now pour in coconut milk, chicken broth with water.
8. Now add sweet potatoes with lime and simmer on low flame. Let to cook for 40 minutes.
9. Garnish with some cilantro.
10. Sprinkle cashews.
11. Enjoy!!

Macros per Serving & Nutrition Facts
- Calories 206
- Total Fat 42g
- Total Carbohydrate 0.5g
- Protein 29g

Coconut Adobo Chicken Stuffed Sweet Potatoes

This dish is packed with unique flavors that you never tried before.

Serving Size: 4
Overall Time: 1 hr. and 30 mins

Ingredients:
- sweet potatoes (3 large)
- chicken breast (3)
- Olive Oil (2 tbsp.)
- salt and pepper, to taste
- bell pepper (1 red, chopped)
- green onions (3, chopped)
- Coconut Adobo Cooking Sauce (1/2 Jar)
- Cilantro (2 Tbsp., chopped)
- Roasted cashews (1/4 Cup)

Directions:
1. Preheat oven to 400 degrees.
2. Rub sweet potato with olive oil.
3. Transfer them to the baking sheet and bake for 1 hour.
4. In a pan heat 1 tbsp. oil and add chicken, salt, and pepper.
5. Cook for about 5 minutes.
6. Now add red bell pepper and green onions, cook for another 2-3 minutes.
7. Add in Adobo Sauce and stir well, cooking for 10 minutes.

8. Cut sweet potatoes as a half and fill them each with chicken mixture, top with cilantro and some cashews.

Macros per Serving & Nutrition Facts
- Calories 305
- Total Fat 16.1g
- Total Carbohydrate 27g
- Protein 15.8g

Fennel Quiche V

This recipe is a remarkably tasty fennel quiche that is healthy as well.

Serving size: 4
Overall time: 33 mins.

Ingredients:
- 10 oz. fennel, chopped
- 1 cup spinach
- 5 eggs
- ½ cup almond flour
- 1 teaspoon olive oil
- 1 tablespoon butter
- 1 teaspoon salt
- ¼ cup heavy cream
- 1 teaspoon ground black pepper

Directions:
1. Chop the spinach and combine it with the chopped fennel in the big bowl.
2. Beat the egg in the separate bowl and whisk them.
3. Combine the whisked eggs with the almond flour, butter, salt, heavy cream, and ground black pepper. Whisk it.
4. Preheat the air fryer to 360 F.
5. Spray the air fryer basket tray with the olive oil inside.

6. Then add the spinach-fennel mixture and pour the whisked egg mixture.
7. Cook the quiche for 18 minutes. When the time is over – let the quiche chill little. Then remove it from the air fryer and slice into the servings. Enjoy!

Macros per Serving & Nutrition Facts
- Calories 249
- Total Fat 19.1g
- Total Carbohydrate 9.4g
- Protein 11.3g

Southwest Tortilla Bake V

This tortilla bake is extremely filling and will keep you full until breakfast the following morning.

Serves: 8
Overall time: 1 hour

Ingredients:
- Whole Wheat tortillas (8, cut in half)
- Monterey jack cheese (1 cup shredded)
- Corn (1 cup, fresh)
- Black beans (1 cup, cooked)
- Green onions (2, sliced)
- Eggs (2)
- Milk (1 cup, fat free)
- Chili powder (1/2 tsp.)
- Green chilies (4 oz., diced)
- Tomato (1, sliced)
- Salsa

Directions:

1. Set your oven to preheat oven to 350 degrees F, and lightly grease a square baking dish with oil.
2. Add 5 tortilla halves onto the bottom of your dish. Top with beans, corn, 1/3 cup of each cheese.
3. Top evenly with a half of your green onions. Top with another 5 halves of the tortillas, then the remaining vegetables, and another 1/3 cup of cheese.
4. Finally, top with your remaining 5 tortilla halves. Add green chilis, milk, chili powder, and eggs then whisk to combine.
5. Transfer your egg mixture in your baking dish and top with cheese. Set to bake until fully set (about 50 minutes).
6. Allow to rest for 10 minutes, then top with salsa, and serve.

Macros per Serving & Nutrition Facts
- Calories 363
- Total Fat 15 g
- Total Carbohydrate 33 g
- Protein 24 g

Washington Apple Turkey Gyro V 20

A Turkey Gyro a basically a turkey wrapped made with a Pita instead of a tortilla wrap. They are delicious and easy to whip up.

Serves: 6
Overall time: 15 minutes

Ingredients:
- Oil (1 tbsp., vegetable)
- Onion (1 cup, thin slices)
- Red pepper (1 cup, thinly sliced)
- Green pepper (1 cup, thinly sliced)
- Lemon juice (2 tbsp.)
- Cooked turkey (1/2 lb., sliced)
- Golden apple (1, finely chopped)

- Pocket pita bread (6, whole wheat)
- Plain yogurt (8 tbsp., low-fat)

Directions:
1. Heat oil in a large skillet over medium heat.
2. Add peppers, onion, and lemon juice and sauté until cook.
3. Mix in turkey and apple and cook until turkey is properly cooked.
4. Remove from flame. Place some of the mixture in each pita.
5. Fill each pita with some of mixture; drizzle with yogurt. Serve warm.

Macros per Serving & Nutrition Facts
- Calories 235
- Total Fat 8 g
- Total Carbohydrate 31 g
- Protein 11 g

Cumin-Spiced Lamb Chops

This Cumin Spiced Lamp Chop recipe will quickly become a favorite event dinner for not only you, but your whole family. To enhance the flavor consider marinating the lamb overnight and allow it to stay chilled in the refrigerator.

Serves: 2
Overall time: 4hr. 40min

Ingredients
- 4 lamb chops
- 2 cloves garlic, mashed
- 2 teaspoons whole cumin seeds
- 2 teaspoons red pepper flakes
- 2 teaspoons coarse sea salt
- 2 teaspoons coarse pepper

- 1 tablespoon olive oil

Directions
1. Preheat the water bath to 140 degrees F.
2. Rub the lamb chops with salt, pepper, garlic, cumin, and red pepper. Seal into the bag.
3. Place in water bath and cook 2-4 hours. Remove lamb from bag and pat dry.
4. Sear on a frying pan with olive oil until brown on both sides.

Macros per Serving & Nutrition Facts
- Calories 200
- Total Fat 13.12g
- Total Carbohydrate 3.96g
- Protein 17.68 g

Dinner Recipes

Tandoori Chicken

This chicken dish has a very specific taste that will entice your taste buds. It's marinated in yogurt and lemon juice then seasoned to perfection.

Serves: 6
Overall time: 35 minutes

Ingredients:
- Plain yogurt (1 cup, nonfat)
- Lemon juice (½ cup)
- Garlic (5 cloves, crushed)
- Paprika (2 tbsp.)
- Curry powder (1 tsp., yellow)
- Ginger (1 tsp., ground)
- Chicken breasts (6 skinless, boneless, cut in strips)
- Skewers (6, soaked in water, then drained)

Directions:
1. Set oven to preheat to 400 degrees F. In your blender, combine red pepper flakes, ginger, curry, paprika, garlic, lemon juice, and yogurt, then process into a smooth paste.
2. Add your chicken strips evenly onto your skewers. Add your chicken to a shallow casserole dish then cover with ½ of your yogurt mixture.
3. Tightly seal, and rest in the refrigerator for about 15 minutes.
4. Lightly grease a baking tray, then transfer your chicken skewers onto it, and top with remaining yogurt mixture.
5. Set to bake until the chicken is fully cooked. Serve, and enjoy.

Macros per Serving & Nutrition Facts
- Calories 177
- Total Fat 7.2 g
- Total Carbohydrate 6 g
- Protein 20.6 g

Turkey Fajitas Bowls 20

Enjoy the Fajita without the wrap. Mexican cuisine can be just as healthy as any other meal you like to enjoy. Here is an easy recipe you can test out for your next dinner.

Serves: 4
Overall time: 20 minutes

Ingredients:
- Turkey breast (½ lb., cut in strips)
- Olive oil (2 tbsp.)
- Lemon juice (1 tbsp.)
- Garlic (1 clove, crushed)
- Chili pepper (¾ tsp., chopped)
- Oregano (½ tsp., dried)
- Bell pepper (1 large, sliced)
- Tomato (1 medium, cut into wedges)
- Cheddar cheese (1/2 cup, shredded)
- Tostada bowls (4 large, warmed)
- Salsa (4 tbsp.)

Directions:
1. Add your oregano, chili pepper, garlic, lemon juice, 1tbsp. olive oil to a medium bowl and whisk to combine.
2. Add in your turkey then toss to coat. Allow to marinate for about 30 min.
3. Set a skillet over medium heat with oil to get hot. Add bell pepper and allow to cook, while stirring, for 2 minutes.
4. Add turkey and continue to cook for about 3 minutes. Add tomato, stir, and remove for heat.
5. Spoon your mixture evenly into your tostada bowls.
6. Garnish with cheese and salsa then serve.

Macros per Serving & Nutrition Facts
- Calories 240

- Total Fat 15 g
- Total Carbohydrate 5 g
- Protein 23 g

Skinny Chicken Pesto Bake

This recipe mixes the delicious flavor of fresh basil with the slight saltiness of parmesan. Serve it with a small serving of mashed potato.

Serves: 4
Overall time: 35 minutes

Ingredients:
- Chicken (160 oz., boneless, skinless)
- Basil (4 tsp., pesto)
- Tomato (1 medium, thinly sliced)
- Mozzarella cheese (6 tbsp., shredded)
- Parmesan cheese (2 tsp., grated)

Directions:
1. Clean, and dry your chicken, then cut into thin strips.
2. Set your oven to preheat to 400 degrees F. Prepare a baking sheet, by lining with parchment paper.
3. Lay your chicken strips on your prepared baking sheet. Top with pesto, and brush evenly over your chicken pieces.
4. Set to bake until chicken is fully cooked (for about 15 minutes).
5. Garnish with parmesan cheese, mozzarella, and tomatoes.
6. Set to continue baking until cheese melts (about 5 minutes).

Macros per Serving & Nutrition Facts
- Calories 205
- Total Fat 8.5 g
- Total Carbohydrate 2.5 g

- Protein 30 g

Spaghetti Squash Lasagna V

It is recommended that you try to avoid process carbs, so you really have to get creative in order to enjoy the meals that you previously liked. Here is one such recipe that gives you a delicious substitute for lasagna.

Serves: 6
Overall time: 1 hour 50 minutes

Ingredients:
- Mariana sauce (2 cups)
- Roasted spaghetti squash (3 cups)
- Ricotta (1 cup part-skim)
- Parmesan cheese (8 tsp., grated)
- Mozzarella cheese (6 oz., part-skim, shredded)
- Red pepper flakes (to taste, crushed)

Directions:
1. Set oven to preheat oven to 375 degrees F and spoon a half of your marinara sauce into a baking dish.
2. Top with squash then top with remaining ingredients.
3. Cover, and set to bake until cheese is melted, and edges brown (about 20 minutes).
4. Remove cover and return to bake for another 5 minutes. Enjoy!

Macros per Serving & Nutrition Facts
- Calories 255
- Total Fat 15.9 g
- Total Carbohydrate 5.5 g
- Protein 21.4 g

Chicken Enchiladas 20

You are going to love this dish.

Serving Size: 2-4
Overall Time: 8 mins

Ingredients:
- Cream of Chicken soup (11 oz.)
- chicken breasts (1 lb.)
- salsa (1/2 cup)
- cumin (1/2 tsp., ground)
- baby lettuce mix (3 cups packaged)
- corn tortillas (4-5)
- cheese (1 cup, shredded)
- cumin (¼, teaspoon)
- chilies (2 green, chopped)

Directions:
1. Transfer chicken to slow cooker.
2. Take a bowl and combine chicken, cumin, soup and salsa. Transfer this mixture to slow cooker.
3. Cook covered for 4- 5 hours.
4. Now shred chicken with two forks.
5. Spread lettuce mix on a platter over tortilla and spread some chicken mixture at the center of a tortilla, roll up. Roll all tortillas in the same direction.
6. Serve and enjoy.

Macros per Serving & Nutrition Facts
- Calories 310
- Total Fat 6.4g
- Total Carbohydrate 2.6g
- Protein 57.9g

Crab Mushrooms 20

These Crab Mushrooms are such a hit! That you will need to make more sooner than you thought.

Serving size: 5
Overall time: 20 mins.

Ingredients:
- 7 oz. crab meat
- 10 oz. white mushrooms
- ½ teaspoon salt
- ¼ cup fish stock
- 1 teaspoon butter
- ¼ teaspoon ground coriander
- 1 teaspoon dried cilantro
- 1 teaspoon butter

Directions:
1. Chop the crab meat and sprinkle it with the salt and dried cilantro.
2. Mix the crab meat carefully. Preheat the air fryer to 400 F.
3. Chop the white mushrooms and combine them with the crab meat.
4. After this, add the fish stock, ground coriander, and butter.
5. Transfer the side dish mixture in the air fryer basket tray.
6. Stir it gently with the help of the plastic spatula.
7. Cook the side dish for 5 minutes.
8. When the time is over – let the dish rest for 5 minutes.
9. Then serve it. Enjoy!

Macros per Serving & Nutrition Facts
- Calories 56
- Total Fat 1.7g
- Total Carbohydrate 2.6g
- Protein 7g

Asian-Inspired Tofu

Many people shy away from eating tofu as it tends to be flavorless if not prepared correctly. Luckily this recipe shows you how to easily pack flavor into your tofu.

Serves: 8
Overall time: 1 hour 6 minutes

Ingredients:
- Tofu (3 lbs., cubed)
- Extra Virgin Coconut Oil (2 tbsp.)
- Garlic (4 cloves, chopped)
- Ginger (2 tbsp., chopped)
- Anise Seed (1 tsp)
- Fennel Seed (1 tsp)
- Coconut Amino (1/2 cup)
- Honey (2 tbsp.)
- Apple Cider Vinegar (2 tbsp.)
- Fish Sauce (1 tbsp.)
- Sesame Oil (2 tbsp.)
- Sesame Seeds (1 tbsp.)

Directions:
1. Put tofu into a large bowl, drain or pat to dry. In a small saucepan heat oil then add garlic, ginger, fennel seed and anise and cook for 3 minutes.
2. Add honey, vinegar, amino and fish sauce and cook for a minute. Remove from flame and add sesame oil.
3. Pour mixture over tofu and stir. Cool and refrigerate overnight, you may occasionally stir as it marinates.
4. Remove tofu from marinade and bake tofu at 375 °until they are done (about 7 – 10 minutes).
5. Remove from heat, sprinkle with sesame seeds and enjoy. Add your favorite side dish or have as is.

Macros per Serving & Nutrition Facts
- Calories 379.2
- Total Fat 20.1g
- Total Carbohydrate 42.1 g
- Protein 13.9 g

Loaded Sweet Potatoes V

Nothing beats a good loaded potato! This recipe uses fresh, healthy ingredients to allow you to have the same delicious flavor associated with a loaded potato without the guilt.

Serves: 4
Overall time: 35 minutes

Ingredients:
- Sweet potatoes (4 medium, roasted)
- Greek yogurt (½ cup, fat free)
- Taco seasoning (1 tsp., low sodium)
- Olive oil (1 tsp.)
- Red pepper (1, diced)
- Red onion (½, diced)
- Black beans (1 1/3 cups, canned)
- Mexican cheese blend (½ cup)
- Cilantro (¼ cup, chopped)
- Salsa (½ cup)

Directions:
1. In a small bowl, mix together your yogurt and taco seasoning well, then set aside.
2. Set a skillet over medium heat with oil to get hot.
3. Add in your remaining ingredient, except potatoes, cheese, and salsa and cook for about 8 minutes or until fully heated through.

4. Slightly pierce potatoes down the center and top evenly with all your remaining ingredients. Serve.

Macros per Serving & Nutrition Facts
- Calories 309
- Total Fat 8 g
- Total Carbohydrate 59 g
- Protein 3 g

Coconut Flour Spinach Casserole V

Low in fat and even carbohydrates; this breakfast recipe is rich in zinc, niacin, fiber, spinach and proteins. You will enjoy this recipe for sure.

Serving size: 6
Overall time: 1 hour

Ingredients:
- 8 Eggs
- ¾ Cup of unsweetened almond milk
- 5 Ounces of Earth Bound chopped fresh spinach
- 6 Ounces of chopped artichoke hearts
- 1 Cup of grated parmesan
- 3 Minced garlic cloves
- 1 tsp of salt
- ½ tsp of pepper
- ¾ Cup of coconut flour
- 1 tbsp of baking powder

Directions:
1. Preheat your air fryer to a temperature of about 375° F. Grease your air fryer pan with cooking spray.
2. Whisk the eggs with the almond milk, the spinach, the artichoke hearts, ½ cup of parmesan cheese. Add the garlic, the salt and the pepper.

3. Add the coconut flour and baking powder and whisk until very well combined.
4. Spread mixture into your air fryer pan and sprinkle the remaining quantity of cheese over it.
5. Place the baking pan in the air fryer and lock the air fryer and set the timer to about 30 minutes.
6. When the timer beeps; turn off your Air Fryer. Remove the baking pan from the air fryer and sprinkle with the chopped basil. Slice your dish; then serve and enjoy it!

Macros per Serving & Nutrition Facts
- Calories 175.2
- Total Fat 10.3g
- Total Carbohydrate 2.4g
- Protein 17.7

Tuscan White Beans with Spinach, Shrimp, and Feta

Veggies and beans go great together. This recipe tosses in shrimp and feta in the combo for a delicious finish.

Serves: 4
Overall time: 25 minutes

Ingredients:
- Olive oil (2 tbsp.)
- Shrimp (1 lb., peeled, deveined)
- Onion (1 medium, chopped)
- Garlic (4 cloves, minced)
- Sage (2 tsp., fresh, chopped)
- Balsamic vinegar (2 tbsp.)
- Chicken broth (½ cup, fat-free, low sodium)
- Cannellini beans (15 oz., no-salt)
- Baby spinach (5 cups)
- Feta cheese (1½ oz., crumbled, reduced-fat)

Directions:
1. Set a non-stick skillet with your half your oil over medium heat.
2. Add shrimp and cook for about 3 minutes (shrimp should be opaque).
3. Remove from heat and set aside. plate. Return the skillet to the heat and allow to get hot.
4. Add sage, garlic, and onion. Stir, and allow to cook for about 4 minutes or until golden.
5. Once golden, add vinegar, stir, and allow another 30 seconds of cooking.
6. Pour in your broth and allow to come to a boil.
7. Once boiling, cook for an additional 2 minutes before adding in your remaining ingredients. Stir, and serve.

Macros per Serving & Nutrition Facts
- Calories 282
- Total Fat 6.9 g
- Total Carbohydrate 22.2 g
- Protein 32.5 g

Cherry Tomatoes Tilapia Salad

Do you want to enjoy a Southern Tilapia salad with easy directions and affordable ingredients? This recipe doesn't need more than a few minutes with flavorful toppings.

Serving size: 3
Overall time: 26 mins.

Ingredients:
- Cup of mixed greens
- 1 Cup of cherry tomatoes
- ⅓ Cup of diced red onion
- 1 Medium avocado

- to 3 Tortilla Crusted Tilapia fillet

Directions:

1. Spray the tilapia fillet with a little bit of cooking spray. Put the fillets in your Air Fryer basket.
2. Lock the lid of your Air Fryer and set the timer to about 18 minutes and the temperature to about 390° F.
3. When the timer beeps; turn off your Air Fryer and transfer the fillet to a bowl.
4. Add about half of the fillets in a large bowl; then toss it with the tomatoes, the greens and the red onion. Add the lime dressing and mix again.
5. When the timer beeps; turn off your Air Fryer and transfer the fish to the veggie salad. Serve and enjoy your salad!

Macros per Serving & Nutrition Facts
- Calories 271
- Total Fat 8g
- Total Carbohydrate 10.1g
- Protein 18.5g

Air fried Radish with Coconut Oil V 20

If you wonder why you should include radishes in your diet, then should know that radishes possess a great pack of vitamin B6, calcium and manganese. This appetizer makes an amazing ingredient that will help boost your digestion and your immunity as well.

Serving size: 3
Overall time: 17 mins.

Ingredients:
- 16 Ounces of fresh radishes
- 2 tbsp of melted coconut oil
- ½ tsp of sea salt

- ½ tsp of pepper

Directions:
1. Preheat your Air Fryer to a temperature of about 400 degrees F.
2. Slice the radishes into thin slices.
3. Place the radish slices in a bowl and toss it with oil.
4. Lay the radishes in the Air Fryer basket.
5. Whisk the pepper and the salt together; then sprinkle it over the radishes.
6. Lock the lid of your Air Fryer and set the timer for about 12 minutes.
7. Set the temperature to about 200° C/400° F.
8. When the timer beeps; turn off your Air Fryer.
9. Remove the pan from the air fryer.
10. Serve and enjoy your air fried radishes!

Macros per Serving & Nutrition Facts
- Calories 148
- Total Fat 14g
- Total Carbohydrate 6g
- Protein 3g

Pork Osso Bucco

This pork recipe goes perfectly with a bit of crusty bread.

Serves: 2
Overall time: 24 hrs. 30 mins.

Ingredients:
- 2 pork shanks
- 1 tablespoon olive oil
- ½ sweet onion, finely chopped
- 1 carrot, finely chopped

- 1 stalk celery, finely chopped
- 4 cloves garlic, minced
- 1 teaspoon salt
- 1 teaspoon pepper
- ½ cup white wine
- oz. whole tomatoes, crushed
- 2 bay leaves
- 2 sprigs rosemary
- 2 sprigs thyme
- Crusty bread for serving

Directions:
1. Preheat the water bath to 175 degrees F. Meanwhile, prepare the sauce.
2. Heat 1 tablespoon olive oil in a saucepan. Add onions, carrots, and celery and cook until onion is translucent.
3. Add garlic and stir. Pour in wine and tomatoes and cook until sauce is reduced and alcohol smell has evaporated.
4. Remove from heat.
5. Season the shanks with salt and pepper. Place each shank into a separate bag and add half the sauce to each bag. Divide the herbs between the bags.
6. Seal and place into the water bath. Cook for 24 hours.

Macros per Serving & Nutrition Facts
- Calories 683
- Total Fat 20.71g
- Total Carbohydrate 18.25g
- Protein 102g

Air fried Okra with Parmesan Cheese V

Air fried okra make one of the best appetizers because it is very low in calories, carbohydrates. This recipe is a perfect choice for people adopting Bariatric diet and it can help boost the level of iron in your blood.

Serving size: 1
Overall time: 35 mins.
Ingredients:
- 1 Pound of fresh okra
- 1 tsp of sea salt
- 2 tbsp of almond flour
- ¼ Cup of finely grated Parmesan cheese
- ½ tsp of pepper
- 1 Pinch of sea salt

Directions:
1. Preheat your Air Fryer to a temperature of about 390° F.
2. Wash the okra; then chop it into small pieces.
3. Toss the chopped okra with the salt and a little bit of ground pepper; then set it aside for about 3 minutes.
4. In a bowl; mix the almond flour with Parmesan cheese, the pepper, and the salt.
5. Coat the okra pieces into the mixture and place it in your Air Fryer basket.
6. Lock the lid and set the timer to about 25 minutes and the temperature to 390° F.
7. When the timer beeps; turn off your Air Fryer. Remove the pan; then serve and enjoy your okras!

Macros per Serving & Nutrition Facts
- Calories 358
- Total Fat 8.6g
- Total Carbohydrate 45.2g
- Protein 24.9g

Vegetables and Turkey Stir-Fry 20

Stir fries are quick and easy to whip up. They are generally filled with whatever you have on hand. This specific recipe uses turkey and mixed vegetables.

Serves: 2
Overall time: 18 minutes
Ingredients:
- Oil (1 tbsp.)
- Salt (½ tsp.)
- Ginger (1 tbsp., minced)
- Garlic (1 clove, peeled, minced)
- Turkey (1 cup, cubed)
- Mixed Vegetables (2 cups, chopped)
- Stevia (½ tsp.)
- Zucchini rice (3 cups, cooked)

Directions:
1. Set a skillet with your oil to get hot over medium heat. When hot, add your turkey, vegetables, garlic, ginger, and salt.
2. Stir-fry on medium for about 2 minutes. Stir in your stevia, then top with zucchini rice.
3. Continue to cook until your vegetables become tender (about another 3 – 5 minutes). Serve, and enjoy!

Macros per Serving & Nutrition Facts
- Calories 183
- Total Fat 9.6 g
- Total Carbohydrate 10 g
- Protein 12.9 g

Spicy Pork Tenderloin with Apples and Sweet Potatoes

Pork and apples generally go together in many recipes. This specific recipe adds potatoes to the mix to create a complete dinner dish.

Serves: 4
Overall time: 47 minutes

Ingredients:
- Apple cider (¼ cup)
- Vinegar (¼ cup, apple cider)
- Maple syrup (2 tbsp.)
- Paprika (¼ tsp., smoked)
- Ginger (1 tsp., grated)
- Black pepper (1 tsp., ground)
- Vegetable oil (2 tbsp.)
- Pork tenderloin (12 oz.)
- Sweet potato (1 large, cubed)
- Apple (1 large, cubed)

Directions:
1. Set your oven to preheat to 375 degrees F. Add your pepper, ginger, paprika, maple syrup, apple cider vinegar, and apple cider in a medium bowl., and use to season your pork tenderloins.
2. Set your Dutch oven with oil to heat up over medium heat.
3. Once hot, reduce heat to low and add pork tenderloins, then allow to brown on all sides for about 8 min.
4. Add in your remaining ingredients around the pork, cover then transfer to oven to roast until pork an internal temperature of at least 145 degrees F.
5. Remove cover, flip potatoes and continue cooking without cover for another 5 minutes.
6. Let stand at room temperature uncovered for 5 minutes before serving.

Macros per Serving & Nutrition Facts
- Calories 339

- Total Fat 12.1g
- Total Carbohydrate 21.3 g
- Protein 35.3 g

Barbecue Ribs

These ribs go best with a fresh garden salad.

Serves: 4
Overall time: 12 hrs. 20 mins.

Ingredients:
- 1 rack pork ribs
- 1 tablespoon salt
- 1 teaspoon pepper
- 2 tablespoons natural stevia
- 1 tablespoon garlic powder
- 1 tablespoon onion powder
- 2 tablespoons paprika
- ½ cup barbecue sauce, plus extra for serving

Directions:
1. Preheat the water bath to 165 degrees F.
2. Combine salt, pepper, stevia, garlic powder, onion powder, and paprika.
3. Rub all over ribs. Seal ribs into bag and place in water bath. Cook 12 hours.
4. When ribs are cooked, place on a baking sheet lined with aluminum foil.
5. Spread barbecue sauce over ribs. Place under broiler until sauce bubbles.
6. Serve with additional sauce.

Macros per Serving & Nutrition Facts
- Calories 579
- Total Fat 19.91g
- Total Carbohydrate 23.99g
- Protein 72.06g

Chicken Cordon Bleu

Enjoy a restaurant quality meal with your family right from your kitchen without the guilt of all the added oil generally required to deep fry a Chicken Cordon Bleu. Enhance the flavor by adding a bit of parsley, thyme, and dried mustard.

Serves: 4
Cook Overall time: 2 hrs.

Ingredients:
- 2 boneless, skinless chicken breasts, butterflied
- 4 deli slices ham
- 4 deli slices Swiss cheese
- ½ cup flour
- 1 egg
- 1 cup bread crumbs

Directions:
1. Preheat the water bath to 140℉. Lay slices of ham on top of butterflied chicken breasts, then lay cheese on top of ham.
2. Trim excess. Roll up chicken breasts with the ham and cheese on the inside.
3. Place prepared chicken breasts inside the bag. Seal tightly and place in water bath. Cook 1 ½ hours.
4. When chicken is done, remove carefully from wrapper and pat dry. Dredge each piece in flour, then dip in egg, followed by the breadcrumbs. Preheat your air fryer to 350℉.
5. Air Fry chicken until golden brown on all sides.
6. Remove to paper towel to drain. Cut breasts in halves, then serve.

Macros per Serving & Nutrition Facts
- Calories 567
- Total Fat 26g
- Total Carbohydrate 34.2 g
- Protein 46.2 g

Lazy Man's Lobster

Consider enhancing the lobster's flavor by testing out other ingredients in the vacuum bag. Fish stock or even brandy can be used, for example, to add an extra punch to your lobster.

Serves: 1
Overall time: 1 hr. 20mins.

Ingredients:
- Tail and claws of 1 lobster
- 2 tablespoons butter
- 1 clove garlic, minced
- ½ tablespoon fresh thyme, minced
- ¼ cup sherry
- ½ teaspoon salt
- ½ teaspoon pepper
- ¼ cup heavy cream
- Toast for serving

Directions
1. Preheat the water bath to 140℉. Seal lobster into the bag.
2. Place in water bath and cook 1 hour. Meanwhile, prepare the sauce.
3. Melt butter in a pan. Add garlic and thyme and cook 30 seconds. Add sherry and bring to a boil.
4. Remove from heat and stir in cream. Season with salt and pepper. When lobster is cooked, remove the shell and stir into sauce. Serve with toast.

Macros per Serving & Nutrition Facts
- Calories 582
- Total Fat 46.26 g
- Total Carbohydrate 5.45 g
- Protein 26.7 g

Grilled Mediterranean Vegetables V

Nothing makes a better snack than a hardy serving of healthy vegetables. Here is a delicious recipe for crispy grilled veggies, Mediterranean style.

Serving size: 6
Overall time: 30 mins.

Ingredients
- 1/4 cup (56 g/2 oz) ghee or butter
- 2 small (200 g/7.1 oz) red, orange, or yellow peppers
- 3 medium (600 g/21.2 oz) zucchini
- 1 medium (500 g/17.6 oz) eggplant
- 1 medium (100 g/3.5 oz) red onion

Directions
1. Set the oven to broil to the highest setting. In a small bowl, mix the melted ghee and crushed garlic.
2. Wash all the vegetables. Halve, deseed, and slice the bell peppers into strips. Slice the zucchini widthwise into 1/4-inch (about 1/2 cm) pieces. Wash the eggplant and slice. Quarter each slice into 1/4-inch (about 1/2 cm) pieces. Peel and slice the onion into medium wedges and separate the sections using your hands. Place the vegetables in a bowl and add the chopped herbs, ghee with garlic, salt, and black pepper.
3. Spread all the vegetables on a baking sheet, ideally on a roasting rack or net so that the vegetables don't become soggy from the juices. Transfer to the oven and cook for about 15 minutes. Be careful not to burn them.
4. When done, the vegetables should be slightly tender but still crisp. Serve with meat dishes or bake with cheese such as feta, mozzarella, or halloumi.

Macros per Serving & Nutrition Facts
- Calories 89

- Total Fat 17g
- Total Carbohydrate 7g
- Protein 14g

Halibut with Chili and Smoked Paprika

Are you ready for a sumptuous and easy dinner? Get ready for a dinner without mess and with a great pack of nutrients. What are you waiting for to enjoy this dinner!

Serving size: 2-3
Overall time: 23 mins.

Ingredients:
- 4 Cups of packed spinach
- 2 Halibut steaks of 11oz each
- The Juice of half a lemon
- 1 Pinch of salt
- 1 Pinch of pepper
- 1 Pinch of smoked paprika
- 1 sliced lemon
- Sliced green onions
- 1 Deseeded and thinly sliced red chili
- 1 Cup of halved cherry tomatoes
- 2 tbsp of avocado oil

Directions:
1 Preheat your Air Fryer to a temperature of 200° C/ 400°F.
2 Lay two squares of the same size of foil over a flat surface. Divide the spinach between the squares.
3 Place the halibut steaks over a chopping board; then remove the membrane and the bone. You should have about pieces all in all.

4   Lay the first 2 pieces of halibut over each of the spinach piles; the squeeze the lemon over each. Season with smoke paprika. Top with lemon slices.
5   Top each fillet with the sliced green onions, the chili and the cherry tomatoes.
6   Pour 1 tbsp of avocado oil over each fish portion.
7   Tightly wrap the foil around the fish; then arrange the two in the air fryer pan.
8   Lock the lid of your air fryer and set the timer to 13 minutes and the temperature to 400° F. When the timer beeps; turn off your air fryer.
9   Serve and enjoy your dinner!

Macros per Serving & Nutrition Facts
- Calories 350
- Total Fat 18g
- Total Carbohydrate 9g
- Protein 43g

Snack Recipes

Un-beet-able Berry Smoothie V 20

This smoothie is packed with protein and naturally sweetened with berries.

Serves: 2
Overall time: 8 minutes

Ingredients:
- Pineapple juice (1 cup)
- Low-fat yogurt (1 cup, vanilla)
- Strawberries (1 cup, frozen)
- Blueberries (1⁄2 cup, frozen)
- Beets (1⁄2 cup canned, sliced, drained)

Directions:
1. Add all your ingredients to a blender, and process until smooth. Serve and enjoy!

Macros per Serving & Nutrition Facts
- Calories 10
- Total Fat 0g
- Total Carbohydrate 1.9 g
- Protein 0.7 g

Strawberry Frozen Yogurt Squares V 20

This homemade yogurt will become one of your favorite snacks if you generally like sweets. It offers you the creaminess of ice cream with the natural sweetness of strawberries.

Serves: 8
Overall time: 8 hours

Ingredients:

- Barley & wheat cereal (1 cup)
- Fat- free yogurt (3 cups, strawberry)
- Strawberries (10 oz., frozen)
- Milk (1 cup, fat-free, condensed)
- Whipped topping (1 cup, fat-free)

Directions:
1. Prepare a baking tray by lining it with parchment paper.
2. Spread your cereal evenly over the bottom of the tray.
3. Add milk, strawberries, yogurt to your blender, and process into a smooth mixture.
4. Use your yogurt mixture to top cereal, wrap with foil, and place to freeze until firm (about 8 hours).
5. Slightly thaw, slice into squares and serve.

Macros per Serving & Nutrition Facts
- Calories 188
- Total Fat 0g
- Total Carbohydrate 43.4 g
- Protein 4.6 g

Smoked Tofu Quesadillas 20

These quesadillas are made from all-natural ingredients and are simply delish.

Serves: 4
Overall time: 26 minutes

Ingredients:
- Tofu (1lb, extra firm, drained, thinly sliced, smoked, grilled)
- Tortillas (12)
- Coconut oil (2 tablespoons)
- Cheddar cheese (6 slices)
- Sundried tomatoes (2 tablespoons)

- Cilantro (1 tablespoon)
- Sour cream (5 tablespoons)

Directions

1. Lay one tortilla flat and fill with tofu, tomato, cheese and top with oil.
2. Repeat for as many as you need. Bake for 5 minutes and remove from flame.
3. Top with sour cream.

Macros per Serving & Nutrition Facts
- Calories 136
- Total Fat 6 g
- Total Carbohydrate 13 g
- Protein 10 g

Tzatziki V 20

This Tzatziki makes a delicious dip for vegetable crudités.

Serves: 10
Overall time: 10 minutes

Ingredients:
- Low-fat yogurt (3 cups, plain)
- Lemon juice (3 tbsp.)
- Garlic (1 clove, finely minced)
- Cucumbers (2 medium, peeled, seeded, grated)
- Dill (1 tbsp., chopped)
- Salt (½ tsp.)
- Black pepper (¼ tsp.)

Directions:

1. Fit a fine meshed strainer with paper towel then pour your yogurt in it and leave to drain over a bowl.

2. Set in the refrigerator for about 2 hours. Transfer yogurt to a large bowl and discard drippings. Add cucumber and salt into a medium bowl then toss to coat.
3. Squeeze your cucumber between paper towels to remove any excess liquid then add to your yogurt bowl.
4. Add your remaining ingredients, and chill in the refrigerator for a few hours before serving.

Macros per Serving & Nutrition Facts
- Calories 50
- Total Fat 1.7 g
- Total Carbohydrate 3.2 g
- Protein 5.2 g

Zucchini Pizza Boats V

These boats make delicious snacks. Fill them with pizza sauce and mozzarella and you got yourself a healthy mini cheese pizza.

Serves: 2
Overall time: 45 minutes

Ingredients:
- Zucchini (2 medium, washed, trimmed)
- Tomato Sauce (1/2 cup)
- Mozzarella cheese (1/2 cup shredded, reduced-fat)
- Parmesan cheese (2 tbsp.)

Directions:
1. Set your oven to preheat to 350 degrees F.
2. Slice your zucchini in half lengthwise and spoon out the core and seeds to form boats.
3. Put your zucchini halves, skin side down in a small baking dish.

4. Add your remaining ingredients inside the hollow center then set to bake until golden brown, and fork tender (about 30 minutes).
5. Serve, and enjoy.

Macros per Serving & Nutrition Facts
- Calories 214
- Total Fat 7.9 g
- Total Carbohydrate 23.6 g
- Protein 15.2 g

Curried Acorn Squash V

This dish is extremely easy to whip up and can act as a filling side dish for just about any entrée you would like. This delicious squash can be served with a variety of additions like refried beans or even a serving of stir fried vegetables.

Serves: 4
Overall time: 2hrs 30 mins.

Ingredients:
- 1 acorn squash, seeded and cut into wedges
- 2 tbsp. butter
- 1 tbsp. curry powder or garam masala
- ¼ tsp. salt

Directions:
1. Preheat the water bath to 185℉ . Combine squash, butter, spice mix, and salt in a bag.
2. Seal and place in water bath. Cook 1 ½ to 2 hours.

Macros per Serving & Nutrition Facts
- Calories 99
- Total Fat 1.2 g

- Total Carbohydrate 12.1 g
- Protein 6.1g

Turkey bacon Brussels Sprouts V

These Turkey bacon brussel sprouts uses the rendered fat from the Turkey bacon to add a dash of flavor to your generally bitter brussel sprouts. To enhance the flavor consider adding a bit of Apple Cider Vinegar and topping with crispy Turkey bacon bits.

Serves: 4
Overall time: 1hrs 25mins

Ingredients:
- Brussels sprouts (1 lb., trimmed, halved)
- 2 tbsp. butter
- 2 ounces thick-cut Turkey bacon, fried and chopped
- 2 cloves garlic, minced
- ¼ tsp. salt
- ¼ tsp. pepper

Directions:
1. Preheat the water bath to 183℉. Combine all your ingredients in a large Ziploc bag.
2. Seal and place in water bath. Cook 1 hour. Meanwhile, preheat oven to 400℉. After 1 hour has passed, transfer Brussels sprouts onto a lined baking tray.
3. Set to bake until nicely roasted (about 5 minutes). Enjoy!

Macros per Serving & Nutrition Facts
- Calories 230
- Total Fat 20.2g
- Total Carbohydrate 10.8g
- Protein 4g

Zucchini Walnut Muffins V

Muffins are delicious! Unfortunately, most muffins are made with all-purpose flour, which makes them taboo for people on the Gastric

Sleeve recovery diet. Luckily, this recipe provides you with an easy zucchini-based recipe that is just as tasty.

Serves: 12
Overall time: 40 minutes

Ingredients:
- Whole wheat flour (2 cup, pastry)
- Cinnamon (½ tsp.)
- Nutmeg (¼ tsp., ground)
- Baking powder (1½ tsp.)
- Baking soda (½ tsp.)
- Slat (¾ tsp.)
- Stevia (1 cup)
- Butter (2 tbsp., melted)
- Milk (¾ cup, low-fat)
- Zucchini (1 cup, shredded)
- Canola oil (2 tbsp.)
- Egg (1 large)

Directions:
1. Set your oven to preheat to 400 degrees F, and lightly grease a 12-cup nonstick muffin tin.
2. Next add all your dry ingredients in a large bowl, then combine all the wet ingredients in a separate bowl, and mix to combine.
3. Pour your wet ingredients into the dry bowl, and fold to incorporate.
4. Divide evenly into your muffin tin and set to bake until fully baked (about 30 minutes).
5. Cool slightly on a wire rack and serve.

Macros per Serving & Nutrition Facts
- Calories 140
- Total Fat 7g
- Total Carbohydrate 18 g

- Protein 2 g

Parsley Flakes Onion Chips V 20

Onion is known for being one of the best ingredients that can help boost your immune system, especially when you are adopting a diet like the Bariatric diet. This appetizing recipe will help you lose weight in a short time as well.

Serving size: 2-3
Overall time: 19 mins.

Ingredients:
- 1 Onion
- 1 Large egg
- 2 Tbsp of coconut flour
- 2 Tbsp of grated parmesan cheese
- 1/8 tsp of garlic powder
- ¼ tsp of parsley flakes
- 1/8 tsp of cayenne pepper
- 1 Pinch of salt
- 1 Tbsp of olive oil

Directions:
1. Preheat your Air Fryer to a temperature of 360° F. Crack the egg and beat it a shallow bowl.
2. Mix the parmesan with the coconut flour, the garlic powder, the parsley flakes, the cayenne and the salt in a shallow bowl.
3. Slice the onion into rings of about ½ inch of thickness. Add the onion rings to the egg wash for about 1 minute; then coat very well.

4. Remove the onion rings from the egg wash; then coat it in the shallow dish of the flour. Arrange the onion rings in the Air Fryer basket; then drizzle with 1 tbsp of oil.
5. Lock the lid of your Air Fryer. Set the timer for about 9 to 10 minutes and set the temperature to about 200°C/ 390° F.
6. When the timer beeps; turn off your Air Fryer. Serve and enjoy your delicious appetizer!

Macros per Serving & Nutrition Facts
- Calories 170
- Total Fat 8.1g
- Total Carbohydrate 12g
- Protein 3g

Whole Wheat Muffins V

These muffins are satisfying and tasty.

Serves: 4
Overall time: 35 minutes

Ingredients:
- Olive oil cooking spray
- Whole wheat flour (2 cups)
- Stevia (1/4 cup)
- Baking powder (3½ tsp.)
- Egg whites (2 eggs)
- Canola oil (3 tbsp.)
- Buttermilk (1 1/3 cups, fat-free)

Directions:
1. Set oven to preheat to 350 degrees F and prepare a muffin tin by lightly greasing with cooking spray.
2. Add all your dry ingredients to a large mixing bowl and set aside.

3. Add all your remaining ingredients to a separate bowl.
4. Add wet ingredients into the dry bowl and gently fold to combine.
5. Transfer batter evenly into your muffin tins and bake until fully cooked (about 30 minutes).

Macros per Serving & Nutrition Facts
- Calories 195
- Total Fat 7.7g
- Total Carbohydrate 28 g
- Protein 5.5 g

Skinny Ranch Dip V 20

Here we have yet another dip that goes well with your veggie crudités.

Serves: 1
Overall time: 20 minutes

Ingredients:
- Mayonnaise (2 tbsp., light)
- Greek yogurt (2 tbsp., fat free)
- Scallion (2 tbsp., chopped)
- Salt and fresh pepper

Directions:
1. Add all your ingredients to a medium bowl, then stir well. Serve, and enjoy!

Macros per Serving & Nutrition Facts
- Calories 140
- Total Fat 14 g
- Total Carbohydrate 2 g
- Protein 1 g

Skillet Granola V 20

This recipe provides a simple granola that you can make on the stovetop.

Serves: 4
Overall time: 17 minutes

Ingredients:
- 1/3 cup vegetable oil
- 3 tablespoons honey
- ¼ cup powdered milk
- Vanilla (1 tsp.)
- Oats (4 cups, uncooked, old-fashioned, rolled)
- Sunflower seeds (½ cup)
- Raisins (1 cup)

Directions:
1. Prepare a baking sheet, by lining with parchment waxed paper.
2. Set a skillet with honey, and oil, over medium heat.
3. When warm, add vanilla, and milk then stir.
4. Next, add in your remaining ingredients, and mix until fully coated.
5. Allow to cook until oats begin to brown, then transfer to baking sheet.
6. Spread that it is flat and allow to cool before serving. Slice and serve.

Macros per Serving & Nutrition Facts
- Calories 210
- Total Fat 8 g
- Total Carbohydrate 28 g
- Protein 5 g

Two Tomato Bruschetta V 20

These Bruschetta are so delicious that you won't want snack time to end.

Serves: 3
Overall time: 17 minutes

Ingredients:
- Feta cheese (1/2 cup, crumbled)
- Tomatoes (1/2 cup dried, chopped)
- Basil (3 tbsp., fresh, chopped)
- Parsley (3 tbsp., fresh, chopped)
- Olive oil (3 tbsp., divided)
- Garlic (2 cloves, minced)
- Black pepper (½ tsp., ground)
- Baguette (12 slices, whole-wheat)
- Tomatoes (3 small, Roma, sliced)

Directions:
1. Set oven to preheat oven to 350 degrees F. Add parsley, basil, tomatoes, and feta to a small bowl, stir and set aside.
2. In a separate bowl, add pepper, garlic, and oil then use it to brush your bread slices.
3. Add your bread to a baking sheet and set to toast for about 5 minutes.
4. Top with your remaining ingredients and set to broil for about 2 minutes to melt cheese. Enjoy!

Macros per Serving & Nutrition Facts
- Calories 57.9
- Total Fat 2.5 g
- Total Carbohydrate 7.9 g
- Protein 1.4 g

Zucchini Pizza Bites V 20

These bites are similar to the zucchini boats, they will remind you of cheese pizza bites.

Serves: 4
Overall time: 11 minutes

Ingredients:
- Zucchini (4 large slices)
- Olive oil cooking spray
- Pepper (½ tsp.)
- Pizza sauce (4 tbsp.)
- Mozzarella cheese (2 tbsp., shredded)

Directions:
1. Set broiler to preheat to 500 degrees F.
2. Lightly grease your zucchini slices with olive oil, then set to boiler for about 2 min per side.
3. Remove from heat then top evenly with your remaining ingredients.
4. Return to broiler and allow to broil until cheese is melted. Serve, and enjoy!

Macros per Serving & Nutrition Facts
- Calories 124.8
- Total Fat 3 g
- Total Carbohydrate 10.4 g
- Protein 8.2 g

Dessert Recipes

Yogurt with Fresh Strawberries and Honey V 20

Yogurt though simple, can serve for a delicious, simple and healthy dessert when topped with fresh fruit. Here is one such simple recipe.

Serves: 4
Overall time: 15 minutes

Ingredients:
- Strawberries (1 pint, fresh)
- Honey (4 tsp.)
- Plain Yogurt (3 cups, low fat)
- Almonds (4 tbsp., toasted, sliced)

Directions:
1. Prep your strawberries, first trim the tops, wash them then slice in halves.
2. Set the strawberries aside. Divide your yogurt evenly into 4 serving glasses, then do the same with the strawberries on top.
3. Garnish each with almonds, and honey then serve. Enjoy!

Macros per Serving & Nutrition Facts
- Calories 262.5
- Total Fat 9.8g
- Total Carbohydrate 38.9 g
- Protein 6.1 g

Pear-Cranberry Pie with Oatmeal Streusel V

These streusels are low in sugar yet still delicious.

Serves: 6
Overall time: 1 hour 30 minutes

Ingredients:

Streusel:
- Oats (¾ cup, regular)
- Stevia (1/3 cup)
- Cinnamon (½ tsp., ground)
- Nutmeg (¼ tsp., ground)
- Butter (1 tbsp., unsalted, cubed)

Filling:
- Pears (3 cups, cubed)
- Cranberries (2 cups, fresh)
- Stevia (½ cup)
- Cornstarch (2 ½ tbsp.)
- OTHER: Pie Crust (1, deep-dish)

Directions:
1. Set your oven to preheat to 350 degrees F.
2. Combine all your streusel ingredients in a food processor and process into a coarse crumb.
3. Next, combine all your filling ingredients in a large bowl and toss to combine.
4. Transfer you filling into your pie crust, then top with streusel mix.
5. Set to bake until golden brown (about an hour). Cool and serve.

Macros per Serving & Nutrition Facts
- Calories 280
- Total Fat 9 g
- Total Carbohydrate 47 g
- Protein 1 g

Lactose-Free Chocolate Pudding V

Here we have a chocolate pudding that is both dairy and sugar free.

Serves: 8
Overall time: 30 minutes

Ingredients:
- Low-fat milk (14 cups)
- Cornstarch (¼ cup)
- Cocoa powder (¼ cup, unsweetened)
- Salt (¼ tsp.)
- Chocolate (2 oz., unsweetened, chopped)
- Stevia (¼ cup + 2 tbsp.)
- Vanilla (1 tsp., pure)

Directions:
1. Combine a half of your milk and cornstarch in a medium bowl and whisk to combine.
2. Set a heavy saucepan over medium heat with your remaining ingredients, stir and cook until chocolate is completely melted.
3. Reduce heat to low and add your cornstarch mixture while whisking.
4. Allow to cook, while stirring for about 10 minutes, or until very thick.
5. Turn the heat off and stir. Allow to cool then stir and transfer to custard cups.
6. Tightly cover, then allow to set in the refrigerator until set.

Macros per Serving & Nutrition Facts
- Calories 157
- Total Fat 4.5 g
- Total Carbohydrate 25.9 g
- Protein 3.1 g

Oatmeal Walnut Chocolate Chip Cookies V

Everyone deserves to enjoy a treat every now and then. These cookies are so tasty you will find it hard to have only one.

Serves: 49
Overall time: 36 minutes

Ingredients:
- Oats (2 cups, rolled)
- Flour (1 cup, whole-wheat, pastry)
- Cinnamon (1 tsp., ground)
- Baking soda (1/2 tsp.)
- Salt (1/2 tsp.)
- Tahini (1/2 cup)
- Butter (4 tbsp., unsalted, cubed)
- Stevia (1 1/3 cup)
- Egg (1 whole + 1 egg white only)
- Vanilla extract (1 tbsp.)
- Chocolate chips (1 cup, semisweet)
- Walnuts (1/2 cup, chopped)

Directions:
1. Set your oven to preheat to 350°F. Prepare 2 sheet pans by lining them with parchment paper.
2. Combine all your dry ingredients and butter in a food processor and process into a crumb.
3. Add in your wet ingredients and continue to process to form a dough.
4. With slightly wet hands roll dough into 49 even balls, add to baking trays and flatten slightly.
5. Set to bake until golden brown (about 16 minutes). Cool then serve.

Macros per Serving & Nutrition Facts
- Calories 160

- Total Fat 8 g
- Total Carbohydrate 21 g
- Protein 1 g

Light and Easy Pear-Strawberry Trifle V

The combination of pears and strawberries in this recipe makes the most delicious trifle.

Serves: 4
Overall time: 30 minutes

Ingredients:
- Pears (2, cored, and thinly sliced)
- Lemon juice (2 tbsp.)
- Strawberries (2 cups, chopped)
- Almond Extract (½ tsp.)
- Orange juice (2 tbsp.)
- Honey (2 tbsp.)
- Angel food cake (½ of a 9-inch cake, cubed)
- Yogurt (3 cups, vanilla)
- Pear slices (1, cubed, for garnish)
- Mint sprigs (3, for garnish)

Directions:
1. Add your salt, stevia, cocoa powder, cornstarch to a medium saucepan, then stir.
2. Add milk, then place over medium heat, while stirring, until the mixture becomes thick.
3. Switch the heat off, then add in your remaining ingredients and whisk briskly until chips are melted.
4. Split your mixture between 4 serving bowls, cover tightly, and refrigerate until fully set. Enjoy!

Macros per Serving & Nutrition Facts

- Calories 210
- Total Fat 8 g
- Total Carbohydrate 28 g
- Protein 5 g

Macerated Summer Berries with Frozen Yogurt V 20

If you were an ice cream lover prior to your surgery you will definitely appreciate this frozen yogurt.

Serves: 4
Overall time: 20 minutes

Ingredients:
- Strawberries (1 cup, sliced)
- Blueberries (1 cup, fresh)
- Raspberries (1 cup, fresh)
- Stevia (1 tbsp.)
- Orange zest (1 tsp.)
- Orange juice (2 tbsp.)
- Yogurt (1-pint, low fat, vanilla)

Directions:
1. Add your stevia, orange zest, orange juice, and berries to a large bowl.
2. Toss to combine. Set to chill for at least 2 hours.
3. Divide your yogurt evenly into 4 serving bowls, top evenly with berry mixture, and serve.

Macros per Serving & Nutrition Facts
- Calories 133
- Total Fat 1 g
- Total Carbohydrate 28.4 g
- Protein 1.3 g

Chocolate Coated Strawberry V 20

This dessert is simple but it is so delicious that you wont believe it wasn't harder to create.

Serves: 10
Overall time: 40 minutes

Ingredients:
- 1 cup raw chocolate minimum 70%
- 10-12 fresh strawberries
- 1 tablespoon butter

Directions:
1. Melt the chocolate with chocolate syrup add butter, leave to cool.
2. Now dip halved strawberry into chocolate mixture and place on platter.
3. Repeat the same procedure for all strawberries.
4. Place the platter into the freezer for 25 minutes. Serve and enjoy.

Macros per Serving & Nutrition Facts
- Calories 98
- Total Fat 1.5 g
- Total Carbohydrate 21 g
- Protein 1 g

Pumpkin Pie Spiced Yogurt V 20

This frozen yogurt will remind you of Thanksgiving.

Serves: 2
Overall time: 15 minutes

Ingredients:
- Low fat Yogurt (2 cups, plain)
- Pumpkin puree (½ cup)
- Cinnamon (¼ tsp.)
- Pumpkin pie spice (¼ tsp.)
- Walnuts (¼ cup, chopped)
- Honey (1 tbsp.)

Directions:
1. Combine all your spices with the pumpkin puree in a medium bowl and stir.
2. Stir in yogurt, divide into 2 serving glasses. Top with honey and walnuts. Serve, and enjoy!

Macros per Serving & Nutrition Facts
- Calories 208
- Total Fat 7 g
- Total Carbohydrate 22 g
- Protein 16 g

The Best Light Pumpkin Pie V

Finally, we have found a pumpkin pie that is low in sugar and made with skim milk yet still as creamy and delicious as you would expect a pumpkin pie to be.

Serves: 8
Overall time: 1 hour

Ingredients:
- Ginger snaps (1 cup)
- Pumpkin puree (16 oz.)
- Egg whites (½ cup)
- Stevia (½ cup)
- Pumpkin pie spice (2 tsp.)

- Skim milk (12 oz., evaporated)

Dlrections:
1. Set oven to preheat to 350 degrees F. Add your cookies to a food processor, and ground to a crumb.
2. Prepare a pie pan (preferably 9-inch) by lightly greasing with cooking spray.
3. Add your cookie crumbs to the pie dish and pat to form a crust.
4. Combine all your remaining ingredients into a large bowl and whisk to combine.
5. Transfer the mixture to your cookie crust and set to bake until fully set (about 45 min).
6. Cool slightly then place in the refrigerator to chill before serving. Enjoy!

Macros per Serving & Nutrition Facts
- Calories 105.6
- Total Fat 0.2g
- Total Carbohydrate 21 g
- Protein 5.5 g

Milk Chocolate Pudding V 20

If you generally love milk chocolate, then this recipe is bound to rock your world.

Serves: 4
Overall time: 10 minutes

Ingredients:
- Cornstarch (3 tbsp.)
- Cocoa powder (2 tbsp.)
- Stevia (2 tbsp.)
- Salt (1/8 tsp.)

- Milk (2 cups, nonfat)
- Chocolate chips (1/3 cup)
- Vanilla (1/2 tsp.)

Directions:

1. Combine all your ingredients, except chocolate, and vanilla, in a medium saucepan over medium heat, while stirring, until the mixture gets thick.
2. Switch off heat then add in your remaining ingredients, and stir until chocolate melts, and pudding gets smooth.
3. Transfer the pudding into 4 serving dishes, wrap tightly, and refrigerate until set. Serve.

Macros per Serving & Nutrition Facts
- Calories 130
- Total Fat 1.5g
- Total Carbohydrate 30 g
- Protein 1 g

Tahini and Almond Cookies V

These cookies provide you with the perfect line between savory hummus and sweet cookies.

Serves: 54
Overall time: 29 minutes

Ingredients:
- Flour (1 cup, unbleached)
- Whole wheat flour (1 cup + 2 tbsp.)
- Almond meal (2/3 cup)
- Butter (½ cup + 3 tbsp. unsalted, cubed)
- Brown (¾ cup)
- Vanilla (1 tsp., extract)
- Salt (1/4 tsp.)
- Water (2 tbsp.)

- Tahini paste (¾ cup + 2 tbsp.)

Directions:

1. Set oven to preheat oven to 350 degrees F and prepare 2 baking sheets by ling them with parchment paper.
2. Combine all your dry ingredients and butter in a food processor and process into a crumb.
3. Add in your tahini, and water and continue to process to form a dough.
4. Transfer to a flat surface and knead for about 2 minutes.
5. Roll dough into 54 even balls, add to baking trays and flatten slightly.
6. Set to bake until golden brown (about 14 minutes). Cool then serve.

Macros per Serving & Nutrition Facts
- Calories 83
- Total Fat 3.6 g
- Total Carbohydrate 11.5 g
- Protein 1.5 g

Conclusion

There you have it! Together we have explored 80 Amazingly Simple Recipes that you can enjoy within the final stage of recovery from a Gastric Sleeve Surgery. We are elated that you were able to stick with us to the end and hope you will consider joining us again when we explore yet another culinary adventure.

Achieving a speedy and successful recovery is vital right now, and we want to continue to help you get there. So, be sure to stick to all the guidelines presented in this book and be sure to leave us a positive review if you enjoyed what you read. Until next time, good luck, and have a speedy recovery.

Made in the USA
Las Vegas, NV
21 May 2024

90196198R00187